Heartfit365

Heartfit365

DAVID BUZANKO

What I wish I knew 30 years ago.

This is not a book for athletes. It is a book
for parents in their 40s who hate the idea of
diet and exercise and have no motivation to
get started. This is a real life story of a father
and his struggle to understand why heart
health really matters. That young lady right
above me on the cover is my daughter and
this is my story, not about losing weight or
becoming a triathlete, it's about wanting
nothing more in life than to be her hero.

I believe that experience gives you better
perspective which leads to better choices, ultimately helping you manage your expectations in life.

The secret to looking good, feeling good and
inspiring others to feel the same, is to eat
less processed foods, sit less and move
more. It should be as easy as it sounds.

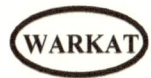

Published in 2014 by

WARKAT Publishing Co.

5 Westmount Court, St. Catharines, ON, L2S4C5, Canada

Buzanko, David, 1966 –

Heartfit365

www.hearfit365.com

ISBN-13: 978-1502925367

ISBN-10: 1502925362

Please consult your doctor before beginning any fitness or dietary program.

Editor: Heidi Geortz

To Robin, Warren & Katelyn

We strive to teach our children about living, but our children have a way of teaching us what life is all about.

The stories that I am about to share are written for my wife, my son and my daughter and for any other parent who believes what I believe.

I believe that quality of life is a choice. I believe that quality of life matters. I believe that being a parent is one of life's greatest responsibilities. I believe that great leaders share two things, they inspire trust and they make those around them feel safe.

What I wish I knew when I was 30 is that food matters, more than you might think. Exercise matters, but not for the reasons you have been led to believe and the biggest reason why any of these things matter is because I want my kids to have a better life than me. I may suffer the same fate as my father, only time will tell. In the mean time I am going to share what I've learned with my kids, if for no other reason than to keep them safe. That's my job as a parent.

Contents

About the Author

Dave Buzanko is a forty-nine year old Long Distance Triathlete, Triathlon Coach, Rowing Coach, Spinning Instructor, Public Speaker, Author, and the Owner of Heartfit365, an indoor cycling studio, as well as Heartfit365.com, an event marketing company that specializes in teaching heart healthy living through employer- sponsored seminars. He has completed the longest triathlon distance in the world at both forty-five and forty-eight years old.

Dave didn't always have all of that athletic street credibility. As a matter of fact, at the age of forty, Dave was just a struggling entrepreneur who found he was tipping the scales at 220 pounds while leading what he considered to be a normal busy and active life, just as most of us do. He considered himself to be no worse off than anyone else living life as a regular "out of shape weekend warrior." Fulfilling his duties and responsibilities as husband and dad, driving to hockey rinks and dance studios, he found the time to squeeze in running his own business and a shift work job at an automotive parts factory.

Like many, Dave found himself facing a midlife health crisis that had been brewing for several years. After a trip to the hospital with chest pains, Dave was faced with a tough decision. He was only forty years old. He could either take control of his health by exercising on a daily basis to manage his heart health and cholesterol, or he could take medication daily, accepting the unknown pathway of declining health for the rest of his life. Dave held many different gym memberships in his thirties, but nothing seemed to be effective. Exercising every day appeared to be his obvious choice, but how could he really do that, and stick with it? What Dave was about to discover was that by changing his focus from losing weight to living heart healthy, he would experience all the difference in the world.

Dave is no different from you. He struggled with diet, exercise and motivation. As you will soon discover, gaining new perspective and understanding the mental side of the decision-making process offered the solutions he had been searching for. It involved consistency, commitment and work. It was the kind of work that you do when no one else is watching. It was more than just weight loss, it was a journey to discover why any of this really matters.

Preface

Today I choose to be heart healthy. Tomorrow I will have to make that decision all over again. I am just an ordinary person who has decided to invest in his heart health every day, and that decision has awakened a new passion for living that I never imagined possible for my life. The only difference between you and me is that today I truly believe that I can do anything that I put my mind to, and I have a system to meet my goals. Making this choice every day does not come without work or sacrifice. If your destination is worthy of the journey and you set your mind on your true motivation and *Why Factor,* then you might just find yourself on this amazing path too.

Every day we are presented with decisions to make and outcomes to live with. As parents in our forties, we spend most of our time thinking about our family's needs and we neglect our own. We put high priority on decisions that affect our kids' health and happiness while giving little or no regard to our own. Of course we all want to be healthy and happy and the two are not mutually exclusive. It's time for some new perspective in your life. It's time to consider all of your

options and the potential outcomes con-
nected to your decisions. On the surface we
may believe we are healthy and happy, because we're used to comparing ourselves to
the people around us. We all live at a certain
level of comfort in our lives, and that is dic-
tated by our immediate surroundings. If you
feel comfortable with your life and yet you
agree with the statement, "I hate exercise
and have no motivation to get started," then
I would argue that you are not happy and
healthy at all, you are simply comfortably
uncomfortable.

As a society, we place a great deal of importance on physical appearances. It's important to us to look good to others, and for
that reason, people will go to incredible ex-
tremes, even undergoing surgery in an attempt to take shortcuts to looking good. It is
our natural tendency to take the easy road
rather than the hard road, and it's clear why
that is the case. The pressure that society im-
poses on us is extreme, so we go to extreme
measures.

Natural beauty is sexier than fake or plastic
beauty any day. There is a certain amount of
confidence and attractiveness that you project when you know you've earned every

pound of the beauty that is your body, re-gardless of your shape or size. Looks can be superficial and are usually trumped by confidence. Real confidence, beauty, and attractiveness come from feeling healthy and acting youthful. I believe that this is the fountain of youth we all go searching for in our forties. Truly, confidence and genuine beauty go hand in hand and they come at a price that money cannot buy. The decision to be confident and beautiful is actually free. The price to be paid is hard work. That is likely to make you feel uncomfortable and even maybe a little bit afraid at first, but with the right plan and the necessary daily motivation, you can live the life you always dreamed and you can inspire others in the process.

Take a look at our North American population. According to a recent study from the American Heart Association, 97 percent of North American adults do not have optimal heart health. Even worse, when polled, over 40 percent truly believed they did. Some of us just know we are not heart healthy but it's the ones who don't even realize it that really motivate me to educate as many people as possible about living heart healthy.

There is an overwhelming need throughout North America for parents in their forties to understand the simplicity and value of maintaining good heart health. Billions of dollars in medical costs could be saved every year if employers understood how to build trust and motivate people.

The premise is simple enough. Help people find their true motivation and then reward them for making healthy choices every day. The upside for the employer is that they will have a healthier workforce with a reduced need for medical care expenses related to unhealthy lifestyles. The benefit for everyone is lower healthcare costs in general, and healthier, happier, and more satisfying lives.

Maintaining great quality of life doesn't need to be costly or complicated. It simply requires a new perspective and the right motivation. Through the internet, you can gain access to coaching and content from around the world. The primary reason why most people are living complacently in an uncomfortable state and accepting that as their reality is because there is no money to be made telling the truth about living heart healthy. Promoting this simple truth is not what makes money for people. There are many companies making billions of dollars selling you machines, advice, dietary programs, pills, and various other kinds of snake oil to turn a profit at the expense of your health. Without a doubt, many companies are offering a valuable product or service, but the real truth is that you don't need to spend thousands of dollars to be happy and heart healthy. What you need is some factual and simple advice, communicated in a forum that everyone with internet capabilities has access to. This book, along with the free content on my website will help you see through the businesses behind the business of the fitness industry. The business behind Heartfit365 are my workshops. This is my opportunity to serve those who serve others. Specifically, parents.

Maintaining good heart health is attainable. It can be as easy as going for a thirty- minute walk every single day and making moderate changes to your diet. The key is learning how to listen to your heart, and you do that by learning to use a simple heart rate monitor.

You certainly don't have to be a triathlete to be heart healthy. Hopefully you will identify with some of my misadventures and glean from the lessons that endurance sport has taught me about life and living to feel alive.

As you learn more about my story, I hope that you will realize that you are not alone in how you think and act. I have shared the same problems as you. The feeling of being alone and helpless to control your heart health and weight can be debilitating. Having an outlet, a good friend, or a mentor like me who will just listen and not judge you is so important to your overall well-being. It's the support that many people simply don't have, yet need, to reduce stress and get on to the road to good health.

I felt isolated for years until I was introduced to my first mentor who, in turn, introduced me to the small community of endurance athletes in my area. These people are unlike your other friends or family. They don't care if your feelings get hurt or if you fail at something; they only care about pushing you to be your better self. They believe in you before you do, and that feeling of unabashed confidence is very empowering.

Access to a good mentor should not be limited to those who can afford literally thousands of dollars a year that some trainers or fitness coaches charge.

Empowering other parents to gain new perspective in their lives and encouraging them to believe that they can make a positive difference in this world is what I have learned to do best.

Nothing can compare to living your life as a heart healthy adult. Your entire outlook on life will change and you will inspire others around you to do the same. Learning how to inspire and motivate others is a selfless act. What you will receive as your reward is a sense of ultimate fulfillment.

You are now the gatekeeper of information. It's up to you to choose to share what you are about to learn. You will learn what inspired me to live heart healthy and you will learn about my daily motivation. More importantly, you will learn that knowledge, just like your belief system, is a very fluid thing.

In triathlon, they say that the first and only goal is to get to the finish line. In reality, my first and only goal is to live my life in a way that helps me look good, feel good and inspires my children.

The Power of One

A chance meeting changed my life forever: five minutes with a complete stranger who shared a common interest and the ability for one of us to step out of our comfort zone and speak up.

Charged with a renewed sense of purpose, I took up the sport of running when I turned forty and consequently ran a minimum of 5k every day for three years straight without taking a day off. I wasn't running all day like Forest Gump did in the movie, nor had I inspired people to join me by covering any great distances. I was simply running 5k to 7k every day, occasionally mixing in the odd 10k for three years. I would later come to understand the benefit of only running these short distances. I was unknowingly doing the right amount of exercise in the right target heart rate zone that allowed me to lose about one pound of fat every month. You have to remember that I wasn't counting calories but I was changing my diet and cutting out a lot of fatty processed foods. This balanced approach to heart healthy living helped me to lose thirty pounds over three years, and at forty-eight, I am now fifty pounds lighter than when I started at forty. I have successfully learned how to manage my heart health and manage my weight through diet and exercise. There is no magic pill that will ever replace the process of making good choices every day that result in the outcome you desire.

One day while I was out for my daily run, I literally ran past an older, silver-haired gentleman who was patiently waiting on his bike for his wife to catch up to him. I noticed he was wearing a tattered old triathlon t-shirt. Clearly it was an old race t-shirt which meant he had probably done that insane distance event. Because he was waiting for his wife, I decided to speak up and ask, "Have you really done that triathlon thing?" As you will discover later in my story, one person with passion and a willingness to share his experiences was all it took to inspire me and change my life forever.

Fast forward two years to age forty-five since that chance meeting and I had completed one full long distance triathlon in Louisville Kentucky, six half long distance races and two sprints. I became the triathlete who started inspiring others. I serve and coach anyone who is brave enough to say "I CAN" and then we simply get on with the process of making that daily decision.

As a guest spinning instructor and rowing coach at the high school level, I have had the opportunity to share my knowledge, story and inspiration with over 2000 high school students and over 1000 adults. While I thought I would be the one inspiring them, quite often the opposite was true.

One day as I was retelling the story of my journey to some of the members at my indoor cycling studio, one of the ladies said to me that the person I had met by chance on the bike sounded a lot like her doctor. I remembered the man introducing himself as a doctor but at the time, I never thought to remember his name. You can imagine his reaction when I arrived at his practice a few months ago to say thank you. I called his secretary to book a five minute meeting and he was extremely shocked and surprised to meet me again and hear how my story had been evolving over the past four years.

I explained to the good doctor that if he hadn't taken the five minutes to inspire me with his story, none of this would have ever happened. I wouldn't be a triathlete. I wouldn't own a cycling studio. I wouldn't have inspired so many people through coaching and I certainly would not have written this book. Most likely, I would have been that guy who tried running and ended up hurting his knees after a few years of a good thing, dropping me into a permanent dependence on heart and cholesterol medication.

Undeniably, one person can make a difference in our world. It's not about standing at the top of the mountain all alone, because as any picture will show you, it's a very lonely place. I'd rather be at base camp inspiring everyone else to believe they can go further in life once they choose to take that next step.

My Story

This part of my story begins when I was turning forty years old. It is likely the part of the book that I believe most of you who are reading it can relate to.

A hockey dad's role changes quickly from making backyard rinks and tying up skates to being banned from the dressing room in just a few short years. Your next role becomes chauffeur and bank machine.

All of the new arenas today have bars in them, so while the kids are at the rink playing hockey, the other dads drink beer and eat bar food to pass the time. In my thirties, I was holding down two jobs, one being a factory job with three rotating shifts and the other was my business. It was not unusual for me to be sleep deprived, and overeating was one way I found to stay awake on midnight shifts.

One cold day in January, just after I had turned forty, I was driving my son to the town of Dunnville for a hockey game. I was experiencing chest pains that simply would not go away. At this point normal people go to the hospital but I waited for the game to end to drive back home before I told my wife what was going on. Rather than suffer the embarrassment of calling an ambulance, I drove myself to the hospital ER. I sat there hooked up to several monitoring devices with three other men in the ward. When the doctor came in, he told me that I had not suffered a heart attack. He knew this because high Troponin levels were not present in my blood work, but I did have high cholesterol and I was most likely suffering from a stress attack. The doctor gave me two choices: lose some weight or go on cholesterol pills for the rest of my life. The choice was mine to make. So I did what most people would do. I stuck my head in the sand and pretended nothing had happened.

About six months after my visit to the ER, I was coming home from buying groceries with my wife and I wasn't feeling too great. I remember thinking to myself that I just wanted to sweat, but in a good way. When we got home I put on my running shoes and went for a 5km run. Truthfully, it was more like a slow jog to the end of my street. I was so winded I had to walk, but I didn't stop. I kept walking and running for the full 5k loop until I got home. I finished what I started.

When I was in my thirties, I had joined a gym and even had a personal trainer and I never lost a single pound. They said I was gaining muscle but I really wanted to just lose weight. My entire focus was on weight loss and that is where most of us go wrong when trying to make improvements to our heart health.

That first day when I decided to go for a run, it wasn't to lose weight; it was to do something good for my heart that day. *My focus had shifted from losing weight to becoming heart healthy*. This was a significant and life-changing shift in my thinking. The next morning I simply decided to get up and do it again.

I hated running as a teenager and I wasn't really keen on the idea as an adult either, but I liked how I felt about myself that day so I decided this was going to be the start of the new me. It took me about three weeks running and walking every day before I could run the entire 5k loop. After about six weeks I decided to sign up for a 5k charity fun run. I had never entered a running race before and I thought it would be a fun new experience to have. I believed that I could run that distance so it seemed like a reasonable thing to do.

I finished that first race and made a video of that experience that you can watch on my Dave Buzanko YouTube channel. After my first race, my friend Michael convinced me to start running a little farther, so I started running 7k every day and we eventually ran in a 10k race together. After three years of running and not taking a single day off, I found myself easily capable of running a half marathon distance on any given weekend.

Remember the story about the older triathlete I met one day while out for my run? It turns out his story was remarkably the same as mine. He had started running when he turned forty for the same reasons but he told me he had turned to triathlon because two of the three sports were non-impact, and should he get hurt running, he would always have the other two to fall back on. That seemed pretty logical. He also told me that in order to finish a full-distance triathlon, I would need to build up my belief system. I would need to learn how to push myself to my limit and then redefine what my next limit would be.

I didn't think too much about that conversation again until a few months later. It was

now November. I had purchased a treadmill
for my wife to use because she had started
running as well, and she didn't like running
in foul weather. I too found myself running
inside like a big baby on days when it was
cold and rainy. This particular day while
running on the treadmill, what did I find on
TV but the triathlon World Championships
from Kona, Hawaii. I remember watching
the guy on TV running, and I was keeping
pace with him on my treadmill. I asked myself, "How hard can this triathlon thing really be?" So when I got off of my treadmill,
I went into my office, got on the internet and
looked up the closest triathlon race I could
find. I didn't even know there were different
distances. I just found the closest event to
me which was the Muskoka triathlon later
that year. The race was about $300 to enter
and I registered right then and there before I
had a chance to change my mind. Then I had
to book my hotel for the event and the host
resort was not cheap. Six hundred dollars
later and I was in this thing for a 1000 bucks
and I had no idea what I was even getting
myself into. I called my wife downstairs to
my office to show her what I had just done.
My recollection of what happened next was
that she looked at me with a kind of puzzled
face, called me an idiot or something to that
effect. But, she was getting a weekend at

Deerhurst Resort so she said, "knock your-self out, I'm in."

The first thing I had to do was learn a little more about triathlons, and my good friend Scott suggested I get a copy of the Triathlete Bible by Joe Friel. I went out and bought this phone book- sized manual and quickly devoured every page. The book made little sense to me, and I was left with more complex questions than I had even known enough to ask. I knew to successfully reach my goal of finishing the race, I was going to need some outside help. A coach!

I was referred to a local coach named Chris and he helped me to make sense of my training schedule for my first year. Chris and I would meet once a week to make sure that I was still on track. It was now January and the race was in early September, so it was time to get started swimming in the pool.

I grew up with a backyard pool and I used to swim in Lake Ontario off of my parents sail boat. I hadn't drowned, so I just assumed I could swim. My son Warren was in grade 10 and his High School had an indoor pool so I brought him along with me on my first day to capture the beginning of my training on film. My kids were fortunate enough to have had private swimming lessons growing up and they were both excellent, fast swimmers.

Do you know who swims in public pools at 7 a.m. in the morning? Right, little old ladies with their flowery swim caps, that's who. I walked onto the pool deck in my brand new Speedo jammers, put my goggles on, ear plugs in and confidently climbed into the water. I started swimming in the outside lane, and about three quarters of the way down the lane I grabbed the wall in a complete panic! I didn't even *know* that I didn't know how to swim. I was devastated! I remember sitting there holding onto the wall and thinking, "what have I done? I've told my wife and all of my friends that I was going to do this triathlon thing and now I am realizing I don't even know how to swim." Warren was dying from embarrassment holding the camera and shouting "just start swimming already, you're embarrassing me." Oh, how the tables had turned.

As I sat there thinking, I just told myself I had to keep going, just like my first day of running. I will never forget what happened next. That little old lady passed me with a very puzzled look on her face and I know what she was thinking: "what an idiot!" It was at that very moment that I learned the first secret to finishing a triathlon; pay your money and tell everyone you are going to do it. You paid your money, you made a commitment and there is no backing out at that point. The only thing left to do was to come back again tomorrow and figure out how to keep moving forward.

It was a choice I had to make every day to keep coming back and swim a little farther just like I did with my running until eventually I would be able to swim the entire 2k distance. It took about two months and swallowing lots of pool water to get there, but I proved to myself again that anything is possible if you simply believe you can.

It was now March and I needed to start thinking about the bike portion of the race. My neighbor Doug had three road bikes and he is about my size. One day I went over to Doug's house and I told him I was going to be doing this triathlon thing and I needed to borrow one of his bikes for a couple of months. He looked me straight in the eyes and said "No." I said "come on, you've got like three road bikes, let me borrow one of them." Again Doug said "No". These aren't triathlon bikes, these are road bikes, what you need is a triathlon bike. You won't be able to run off of the bike if you use one of these. "What the heck is a triathlon bike?" I remember thinking to myself. So off to the bike store I went.

I have never owned a road bike in my life and I had an idea they might be expensive, but I had no idea what I was about to discover. Triathlon bikes start at about $2,200 and go up to about $20,000. After suffering the sticker shock, I ordered my entry level Trek Triathlon bike. I was now into this race for about $3,300. Feel free to insert the word idiot right about here again. That's what I felt like. What started as a $300 race had quickly escalated to over $3,000 and I still needed a triathlon race suit, bike helmet, bike shoes and PEDALS! Yes, all that money and the bike didn't even come with pedals!

I took some deep breaths. I did not have this kind of money to be spending on my new hobby. I was in no man's land. I managed to pull together the money to purchase the equipment and that was not an easy thing to do. My parents actually contributed $1000 towards the new bike. They called it a birthday and Christmas gift rolled into one. I have to give them credit because they don't normally spend that kind of money on gifts

but they did what I would do for my kids.
They just helped because they could.

Three weeks after I got my shiny new bike, I
was out for a ride, and as bad luck would
have it, was hit by a car. I was dressed like a
rolling stop sign: Red bike, red shirt, red
helmet, but the guy driving the car never
saw me. Luckily for me it was a small car,
and I flew right over the hood, across the
windshield, and landed on the road. It was
what I would later describe as the best pop-
up slide of my baseball career. I escaped serious injury with only some scrapes, bruises
and a little road rash. My bike was scratched
up a bit from the impact of the unfortunate
crash to the roadway. The silver lining to the
story was that I wasn't hurt. Because I was
fit, I was able to react and move my body in
a way that I could absorb the impact and roll
off the pavement with minor scrapes and
bruises. My bike was still rideable and the
driver's insurance company bought me a
second brand new bike, so I was on my way
again.

With June quickly approaching, it brought
with it the new challenge of open water
swimming. I grew up with the movie *Jaws*.
We all did. I know it makes no logical sense
to worry about sharks in fresh water, but I

had been scarred for life by that stupid movie. Open water swimming is completely different from pool swimming. You are going to hyperventilate a lot in the beginning and the real trick is to learn how to relax and swim when things are bumping into you or hanging off of you in the water. This is the mistake that most new people make to the sport of triathlon, they don't work on the mental things that bother them the most and they end up entering the water mentally unprepared.

Race day is a very cool, very exciting, and very surreal experience. Once you do any distance triathlon, you are part of the club, a community of adults who come in all shapes, sizes and ability. The only common thread between them is that they all believe they can do anything they put their minds to.

I was ahead of schedule with my training and my coach suggested that I enter a local triathlon race as a warm up to my big September race. Looking back, it was a great decision. As this was my first race, it was very emotional for me. I posted a time of 6:30 and my friends and family were at the finish line to meet me. It's the only race finish my dad has been able to see in person and that left me a little choked up at the finish line. I remember thinking after the race that that was the hardest thing I had ever done because it was very difficult both physically and emotionally. It was a great practice race for Muskoka though, and that experience helped me to have an even better race day in September. My first triathlon distance race was half the distance of a full triathlon and it is all captured on film and you can view it on my YouTube channel. The race in Muskoka was an eye opening experience to the half triathlon distance and the big branded race series. I really knew nothing about the sport of triathlon in the beginning. What I did learn after my first race season was that triathlon is like no other sport in the world. Weekend warriors are allowed onto the same playing field as the pros and you won't find that in any other professional sport. The male and female World Champions were in my race and I stood right beside Mirinda Carfrae (two time World Champion) on the beach by the starting line and I had no idea who she was at the time. That's the beauty of our sport. No pretentiousness, just a simple respect between athletes for anyone who is brave enough to stand at the starting line and say, "I can."

The next season, I set my sights on a full-distance triathlon race in Louisville, KY. Full-distance races typically sell out a full year in advance of the race .This is a very positive thing, because once you make your commitments and pay your money, there should be no looking back.

The good news is that for most people, the easiest way to reduce the risk of many heart related diseases is simply walking, not having to do a triathlon. My story is just that; mine. I haven't shared it with you to brag or boast. I simply wanted to paint a picture for you of how someone who looked pretty good on the surface could have so much going wrong under the hood. If you can glean anything from this part of my story, I hope it is that we all need to step back every once and a while and take stock in our own lives. Look at what you are doing from a new perspective. Look at the decisions you make every day and ask yourself are they really the best choices? Finally, what will your story look like over the next ten years of your life? What will your outcome be? Will you be better off than you are today? I've got news for you: you can be.

140.6 Miles in Seventeen Hours or Less

"Are you crazy? I can't do that, I'm not like those people. I'm way out of shape and way too old." One hundred forty point six miles is the distance you have to travel by swim, bike, and running to complete a full-distance triathlon. There are time cut offs for each event and you have seventeen hours to finish your race. Just for reference, the professionals do it in eight hours.

Why is it that our first and natural reaction to most of the challenging things in life is to start off by saying "I can't," and then stop before even trying? I guess I'm lucky because I stumbled into signing up for my first triathlon based on a chance meeting and not really understanding what I was really getting myself into. Had I known any better, I probably would have said "I can't" as well, and this story would not have had such a positive ending.

My first full long distance triathlon took place in Louisville Kentucky, August 2011. "Swim 2.4 miles, bike 112 miles, run 26.2 miles, brag for the rest of your life," said

John Collins, Ironman Co-Founder. Sounds like fun, right? Did I mention you will likely lose twenty pounds of water weight and burn 13,000 calories or more in one day? You will get nauseated, your butt will get really sore, and you'll question your reason and ability to go on. This is what I experienced during my first Iron distance race and I keep coming back for more.

Spectators play a huge role in helping you mentally get through the race. They make up all kinds of signs for you to read along the racecourse and some are definitely funnier than others. One girl was holding a sign that read, "I don't do triathlons, I do triathletes." An even better sign was being held by a woman near the start of the marathon. We left the transition area to start the run and crossed over a bridge in Louisville that spanned the Ohio River. Coming off the bridge, she was holding a sign that read, "You still think this was a good idea?" Clearly this was a personal message for someone she knew, but I remember questioning myself as if she were speaking directly to me.

We all fear the unknown. Maybe it's the psychology of fight or flight that leads us to naturally being risk averse, but fear is just that, a thought process that we allow to simmer and stew in our gut. It's easier to say "I can't," knowing that others who also fear the unknown will accept that answer because it sounds safe and reasonable. Other people understand how you feel. At one point or another they have felt the same way you do now and are likely to say "I couldn't do that either," so being risk averse sounds like a reasonable plan to them.

What I've discovered is that it is common for people to fear what they don't know. I didn't know that I didn't know how to swim, so when I jumped in feet first, literally, I didn't already believe I couldn't do it. I had grown up with both a boat and a pool and hadn't drowned yet, so I figured I knew how to swim. People generally fear the loss, process, or outcome of risk. Consequently, they spend their entire lives avoiding it, in silence, wondering what might have been. This way of thinking has got to change if you want to experience living healthy, happy, and alive.

Your world and your perspective will dramatically change when you start off a statement with "how can I?" as opposed to "I

can't." When I signed up for my first triathlon, I really didn't know what I was getting
into but I kept saying to myself, "how can I
get through this?" and the answers just
came.

So why do normal, reasonable people take
on challenges like long distance triathlons
and marathons? You might think that people who participate in these events are well
seasoned athletes. You would be surprised
to find that most of the "Age Groupers,"
(these are what athletes are called who are
not competing for prize money), are regular
folks just like you and I who have decided to
take on the challenge for a variety of different reasons.

There are many different types of endurance
races and they are held all over the world.
However, not everyone aspires to be an endurance athlete. Some people handle their
midlife crisis (turning forty) by going on a
special vacation, buying or restoring a car,
or making changes in their personal relationships. I think people tend to do these things
because they want to feel youthful again
while they have the financial resources to
help them feel that way.

But what if you don't have the resources to buy momentary happiness? Is happiness a commodity to be bought or sold anyway? I have many friends who have ample resources but for all of their money they can't buy the experiences I've had. One of my favorite professional triathletes has often been quoted as saying that a full-distance triathlon keeps you honest. Finishing that race is one of those experiences in life that money can't buy, it has to be earned. She's absolutely right, that's what makes it special. If it were easy, everyone would be doing it, and as awesome as that would be, these innovators, would simply move on to something else that offers an even greater exclusivity to membership.

While the name "Ironman" is the brand name of a specific race series, it also depicts a specific race distance, much like an Olympic, Sprint or Tri-a-tri distance. There are many full-distance triathlon races held around the world and some can offer exceptionally difficult challenges.

A good friend and training partner of mine has been working in Finland for the past two years and has discovered a full triathlon distance race in Norway that sends shivers up and down my spine. The race is called the Norseman and what scares me the most is simply realizing that the race exists. The temptation of tackling such an event is very real in my mind. For some reason my spirit keeps telling me this would be a very cool fiftieth birthday present to experience. While my spirit says one thing, common sense or maybe simply fear keeps telling me something else. Fortunately your brain works independently from your spirit and that's how great achievements are accomplished. There are not enough words to properly describe this race so I encourage you to search the Norseman triathlon on YouTube and witness endurance sport in its rawest form. People who take on some of life's greatest challenges are fully aware that the experience they are after cannot be bought or sold. It can only be experienced through years of training along with sheer will and determination, and there is no guarantee that you will ever realize your dream of crossing that finish line.

So what does it really feel like to cross the finish line of a full-distance triathlon? When I did my first full-distance race I went searching for happiness and thought that somehow finishing that race would transform me in that one moment in time and I would forever feel happy and filled with a sense of eternal pride. I ask one simple question of everyone I know who has finished a full-distance triathlon, "Did you go there looking for something and if so, what did you find?" The answer is almost always the same. The average Age Grouper goes in search of that personal moment of glory, the feeling that you simply can do whatever you set your mind to. You do experience that feeling of complete satisfaction when you finally cross that finish line but the moment quickly passes and you're left with another more haunting question... "Now what?"

The "now what" question is the single biggest mental barrier to living heart healthy. If you only focus on weight loss and you are successful at losing your target weight, the question "now what" can stop you dead in your tracks. If however you are focussed on the process of investing in your heart health every day, you answer the "now what" question by investing in your heart all over again tomorrow and the next day. Living heart healthy is like enjoying ice cream, there are so many flavors to experience.

Running down the finishing chute towards the finish line of any full-distance triathlon is absolutely awesome. Where else would you find 5000 people willfully cheering for you to cross a line symbolically drawn in the sand or across a strip of pavement? You're not likely to be in first place and the cheers just keep getting louder the longer it takes you to finish. The crowds continue to grow as more and more athletes finish the race and come back to cheer you in. I have never experienced anything in life quite like it. It is a very humbling moment and when you stop to reflect on what it took to get you there, it's hard not to shed a tear on two. The music will be blaring, the crowd noise will be deafening, and if you are finishing in the darkness of night, you will have the flood-lights shining in your eyes. You will think of your family and the sacrifices they have made that have allowed you to be there and you will search the crowds for those familiar faces.

The reality of the situation is that your family has no idea where you are on the race course. You give them your estimated finish time but anything could happen and they could literally be waiting hours for you to finish your race. Your family is more than likely scouting out the best place to capture that perfect finish line picture before rushing down to meet you after your race is over.

If you're really lucky, the official commentator at your race will have enough time to read your bib number and call you in by name while stirring the crowd into a frenzy. It's an unbelievable rush! Then, just as quickly as the finish line appears, you have your medal around your neck and if you don't require any further medical assistance, your day, your moment and your experience are over. All you have left is the blur of the memory of a day that has gone by so quickly.

Surprisingly, I wasn't particularly sore after my first full-distance race. I was able to walk back to the hotel to take a shower and then walk back to the finish line to rejoin the crowd. I had made a few novice mistakes during the race that cost me over two hours of time and I was thinking more about how I could have been better rather than focussing on being happy and enjoying the moment. I think that was my first indication that I could help inspire and coach others because I was more concerned about the process of perfecting performance than I was about basking in the glory of the moment.

Making mistakes is part of the learning process. Learning from your mistakes makes you a better competitor and coach. I made two major mistakes during my race. I underestimated how the heat and humidity would affect my ability to eat during the bike portion of the race and I was relying on solid energy bars for fuel. After five hours of riding in the heat and humidity, I could no longer tolerate the food I was relying on to get me through the race. Everything on my bike was warm (both food and drink) and I rode the final two hours slow, nauseated, and dehydrated.

I am a very visual person and I learn best by looking at pictures and diagrams rather than reading instructions. When I did the race in Louisville, I looked at the run course and assumed it was a one loop course. As I was approaching what I thought was the end of my day, I turned up the speed for a quick finish. I must have been delirious at this point because I thought I had a sub three hour marathon time going and simply couldn't believe it, and for good reason.

As I approached the finishing chute, there was another runner running beside me. As I entered the chute, suddenly I found myself running alone. I asked one of the volunteers where that man might have gone and she replied "did you do your second loop?" I had heard rumors of a victory lap and for the moment I chuckled with the crowd, turned around and headed out for what I thought was a run around the block.

Before I knew it I was back out on the main run course and heading into a second full lap. I HIT MY WALL! I was angry at myself for not paying attention to the details and for wasting all of that energy on my first big finish. What I thought was a great run time was actually my slowest time for a half marathon distance. I was deflated, but not defeated. I realized I could walk from this point on and I would still finish so I decided to walk for about an hour. It took me that long to stop feeling sorry for myself. Let me tell you it is much harder to start running again at this point in the race once you realize your muscles are beyond being just sore. It takes time, but once you get over yourself and mentally get back to finishing the race properly, your legs start moving faster and you finish what you set out to do in the first place: finish the race smiling.

Two years later, my second full-distance triathlon race at age forty-seven was in Cozumel, Mexico. It was quite a different experience because I went into it with the knowledge and experience from my race in Louisville. This time I went to race, not just to finish. I ended up with a personal best time of 11:25 (two hours faster than Louisville) and my body did pay a price the second time around.

I was fitter and I was prepared with a better race strategy for fuel which allowed me to go faster and push myself harder resulting in a great time and a healthy new respect for anyone who finished ahead of me. After the race was over, my legs started to seize up, and the next three days were spent resting and recovering with very little walking. Recovery though is a very funny thing. I went from needing help to walk on Monday to playing ice hockey back home four days later. Again, I am always astounded how resilient the human body is. My body was simply going through the natural recovery and healing process.

I came to race better prepared and I was paying attention to everything this time. My wall on this day came on kilometer 31 between aid stations when my sodium levels dropped too low and my right hamstring balled up in a severe muscle cramp. This was the most intense cramping I have ever experienced in my life. There were no warning signs, it simply came on with one single stride. I went from having a near perfect race day to being dead stopped in the street.

If I even tried to lift my foot off of the pavement, my hamstring, calf and foot all immediately cramped at the same time. If I had not been prepared and done my homework, my day could have ended right there but I was ready. I had brought five salt tablets and two flasks of cola as back up fuel in the event of cramping. Because I understood my body better and learned from my past mistakes, I was prepared. I faced my wall on that day head on, and within two minutes of taking my first salt tablet, I could slowly walk again. Fifteen minutes later I took a second tablet and within five minutes of that I was back to my full stride. I realized that my old way of training wouldn't work and that being better prepared was part of a winning strategy. What could have been a race ending moment became one of my greatest success stories on that day.

In Louisville, I went searching for happiness by attempting to finish a full-distance triathlon. Within an hour of what was years in the making I was already being hard on myself and questioning my ability to do better next time. NEXT TIME! Are you kidding me? I was more messed up after finishing this race because I didn't find what I went looking for and I wasn't sure I had it within me to do it all over again. There is a reason most people don't take on the challenge of a full-distance triathlon, and that's because it's bloody hard! As you can see though, I did go back with different goals, a different mindset and a better plan and that made all of the difference.

After Louisville, I did two half -distance triathlons and improved my times considerably from previous efforts. I was still learning about the sport, trying to understand how my body and mind could work more efficiently. I was getting faster and my confidence was growing. Enough time had passed and the pain of the process of racing that distance was history. All I could remember was how great an experience it really was.

Some people immortalize their experience by getting a finisher tattoo. Among athletes, opinions vary greatly about getting a race branded finishers tattoo. For me, it symbolized all of the really difficult training days I had, like riding four hours in a downpour convincing myself I needed to have that experience in my memory banks to draw from on race day. I am not a big fan of tattoos in general and I know I would not be happy if my kids came home with a tattoo so I was walking a fine line of hypocrisy when I decided to get mine. My simple analogy to my teenage kids was this: you decide to do something so monumental in your life and you feel that much pride that you choose to brand yourself with ink, please do it tastefully and accept any of the consequences.

I have my tattoo on my right calf. It gets noticed by strangers all the time and my kids always tease me that I wear shorts in cold weather just to show off my tattoo. On a recent family vacation to Mexico, I was playing beach volleyball and when the teams were being picked, I didn't feel like I was an old man trying to look young on the beach. I felt a genuine sense of youthfulness.

One day I was waiting in line at the bank and a little old lady said, "What's that on your leg?" I turned around and told her politely that it was a triathlon finisher tattoo. She looked at me and said "that's crazy." I said, "Getting the tattoo or doing the triathlon?" She smiled and said "both".

I'm very proud of how I turned my health and life around in my forties. This was no easy feat as you can imagine. I will admit that I partially got lucky and did all of the right things for all the right reasons and fate played a hand in many of my experiences. The good news for you is that I was smart enough to pay attention and make some notes along the way. It has taken me seven years of living in my forties as a parent going from an inactive lifestyle to one of an endurance athlete. I guess if you want to put a label on it that makes me an expert on how to survive and thrive as a heart healthy parent in your forties.

I'm particularly thankful of the fact that this experience wasn't dismissed as a mid-life crisis by my family or by me. I remember one specific evening waiting to pick my daughter up from the dance studio when I was just beginning to train for my first triathlon. Another parent and lifelong friend of both my wife and I was at the studio and he looked at my wife and said quietly, "don't worry; it's just a mid-life crisis. He'll do this one race and it will all be over."

I wasn't offended by what he said because for all we knew, he could have been 100 percent right. However, it remains with me, and I draw on that memory whenever I need to remind myself of why I train like I do. I simply refuse to accept that this is just mid-life crisis. It's a daily decision that I make for myself and I choose to invest in my heart health every day. Training for triathlons just makes all of the heart healthy exercise fo-cussed and more fun.

When you start participating in any endur-ance sport, the first thing you notice is that there are no age barriers to participating in these types of events. One of my fondest moments from my first triathlon was during the run portion of the race. I was about three kilometres from the finish when I passed a sixty-seven year- old man. You know the other competitor's ages because they write your age on your right calf. It helps the other racers identify how old the racer is in front of you in case you want to chase them down and beat them in your age group. What stuck with me at that moment was that this man started after me (his age group started after mine) so he passed me at some point and it took me about six hours to chase him down. I congratulated him for the example he was setting and let him know that he was an in-spiration to me before I continued on to the finish line. At that moment my perception of what old age looked like completely changed forever.

My journey has taken me into high schools as a guest instructor where I teach students about triathlon and the importance of daily heart health. I know that most of what I'm saying is lost on these kids, but one day, when I'm racing in my sixties and seventies, I'm looking forward to the day when some young forty- something kid runs up on me and says "hey, I remember you. You're that crazy guy who came to my school and introduced me to triathlons." Who knows, they might even have read my book and used my coaching services all those years later. To me, that would be deeply rewarding.

As you continue to read through this book, I want you to consider the power in the self-affirming words "I can" and "it's possible." The next time you catch yourself thinking or saying "I can't," do something: turn it around and rephrase the statement to *"how can I?"* Starting a sentence with these three simple words has the potential to change your life forever.

Surviving 140.6 miles requires only two things...the belief that anything is possible and being brave enough to say "I CAN."

Being Prepared

In December 2013, I completed my second full-distance triathlon race in Cozumel Mexico finishing with a time of 11 hours and 25 minutes. That's a full two and a half hours faster than my race time was in Louisville two years earlier. Why such a big difference in time? I am getting older and that is supposed to mean slower, right? Being prepared simply means learning from past experiences so that the choices you make while training are designed to improve your outcome.

Earlier in my business career, I had the opportunity to meet with Walter Gretzky on several occasions and was fortunate enough to be interviewed together with him on a local lifestyle television show.

During the interview, Walter shared a few stories about his son Wayne that may have surprised a few viewers. Walter noted that in his youth, while Wayne was a standout player, where he really excelled was in his preparation and approach to playing the game. Wayne was responsible for taking care of his own equipment. That meant taking his equipment out to air dry after every practice or game and going through his mental checklist as he repacked his bag before leaving home again. Wayne was meticulous about this ritual and even as a young boy, being prepared before he left home gave him the confidence and clarity of mind to focus on the job at hand which was being two steps ahead of the play that was about to develop on the ice. Wayne was simply better prepared than everyone else and that was one of the greatest secrets to his success.

I can remember driving my own son to hockey arenas for games on school nights that were up to a two hour drive away from home. Almost inevitably before every game, one of the parents would be blowing a gasket after discovering skates or gloves were still sitting on the laundry room floor back at home. If you've ever been a hockey parent or dance mom, you know that look (if looks could kill). Invariably, that mood would simmer during the game and would usually lead to a very long and unpleasant car ride home. This was a ride that no one ever wanted to be a part of.

We all make mistakes. That's part of the learning process of being a parent. Failing to learn from your mistakes is what separates good parents from great parents.

I made a few key mistakes in Louisville, and part of my training for Cozumel included better preparation for my upcoming race. Learning how to better manage my fuel on the bike, along with a planned rest room stop half way through the bike course, produced a personal best time. On the run, I came in with a completely new race plan because, unlike my first full-distance race, my goal wasn't to simply finish, it was to post a time that could possibly qualify me for the World Championships in Hawaii.

Being prepared not only meant doing the right training throughout the year, it meant carrying the right back-up fuel on the race course. By the time my race in Cozumel came around, I had a much better understanding of my body and how my body consumed food for fuel. This understanding became very specific as I learned more about what food options would be offered at the aid stations on the run course. I knew that in order for my body not to "BONK" or shut down on me on the run, I was going to have to manage and make better choices for my food consumption.

As I will mention later in my food section, during my training I had switched from drinking water from my fuel belt to drinking flat cola. People drink water to stay hydrated but it is an empty fuel source. Running longer, faster, and harder meant I was going to have to fuel my body differently. Flat cola is what is offered on every marathon run course and it was worth investigating why. It seems that dextrose which is the main sugar source in cola is one of the fastest absorbing sugar sources for your body. So when your body needs sugar (glycogen) in the blood stream to perform, flat soda is an excellent option. Cola is not the best option when you are not competing so please keep that in mind as you choose your other drink options to stay hydrated during the day.

I also knew that I would need to consume 300 calories of carbohydrates and between 900 mg and 3000 mg of salt an hour depending on race day weather conditions and my own personal sweat ratio. As an amateur athlete, it's difficult to get a handle on these exact numbers without having access to continuous test results. Only the pros and excessively wealthy athletes can justify having access to this type of data.

Doing my homework and having the basic knowledge of recognizing the symptoms of how my body responds to salt depletion and being prepared to handle it when your sodium levels are getting too low was one of the things I was most proud of in my Cozumel race.

I ended up sixty-sixth for my age group out of over 300 athletes and 565 out of 2500 entrants in the race. Not bad for an old guy who was scared of sharks and couldn't even swim one length of a pool four years ago. As it turned out, I was out of a roll down slot for the World Championships but that wasn't what really mattered. I have become a better triathlete and coach for having gone through the experience and I believe that experience will help me to serve others. It's really hard to teach people about things you haven't experienced firsthand but it comes very naturally when you can share your stories with passion.

If you commit yourself to learn from your experiences you will always be improving your perspective, whether in sport, business, or any other worthy endeavor. The choices you make because of your age and ever growing maturity will help to skew more favorable outcomes in your future.

Being Selfish

To finish any full-distance triathlon for the first time, you have to be selfish. Ultimately, until you cross that finish line, you're really not sure if it's going to happen. Anything can go wrong on race day and until you cross that line, you try to control everything you possibly can to ensure your desired outcome.

When I say anything can happen, I mean just that. My race in Louisville was a time trial start. The athletes began lining up at the swim start at 5 a.m. for the 7 a.m. official race start. My son Warren and I left our hotel at 5 a.m. to head over to the transition area for a final pump up of my bike tires and set up all of my fuel needs on the bike. After everything in the transition area on my bike was prepared to my satisfaction, we headed over to the swim start which was about a half mile walk away to a park known as the Great Lawn. Once your bike is ready to go and any last minute details are taken care of, all athletes are instructed to head over to the Great Lawn for body marking. Here you will find the volunteers who write your race number on your arm and your age on your

right calf so that the other racers and race officials can identify who you are and which
age group you are racing in.

After we passed through the body marking
area, Warren and I proceeded to line up for
the race. The athlete lineup twisted, turned,
and snaked through the Great Lawn for what
seemed like miles. Warren was with me to
hold my spot if nature called and I had to
make one or more trips to the portable out-
houses. At about 6:30 a.m., race officials
started to weed out family members from
the line and I found myself much closer to
the entry point into the water. Nervous energy among the athletes was starting to grow
as we waited in the growing humidity. The
anticipation was almost tangible.

At 7 a.m., the last strains of the National An-
them faded away, and the horn blasted. The
elite athletes were off, followed by a steady
stream of Age Groupers jumping off of the
docks into the water, one after another, like
lemmings. The race organizers were using
the first two boat slips of the local marina as
the official starting point for the race and our
swim course took us out through a narrow
canal that served as the gateway from the
small marina out to the Ohio River. As I
made my way onto the main dock and the

entry point for the race, I had to pass the sheriff's boat house, I noticed one officer scrambling up the dock ramp, passing me with a considerable look of panic about him. I thought nothing of that moment again until we arrived back home and a friend told me that they heard on the news that a local gentleman had died during the swim portion of the race. When I mentioned this to my wife, she said that about thirty seconds after I entered the water, the race organizers stopped athletes from entering the water for about a minute while they helped to get another athlete out of the water who was in distress. I actually remembered seeing a commotion with a group of swimmers hanging onto a paddle board and at the time I just thought that these athletes were all having panic attacks. I remember being surprised at how so many of them could be so mentally unprepared for the open water swim.

Only upon returning home did I realize that a man from Buffalo in his forties, just like me, had started the race, only to experience a panic attack in the middle of the pack of swimmers, and shortly thereafter, he suffered a fatal heart attack. When I retell this story to people I coach, I ask them to look around at what thirty people exercising close together looks like and then I ask them to imagine 2000 people all swimming to the same place with limited visibility in the churning water. Sometimes bad things happen to good people. The outcome for this racer and his family was definitely not what he expected it to be.

One of the ways we can prevent the fear of bad things happening to us is by being as prepared as we can possibly be and this is where the controlling and selfish behavior begins to creep in. On one hand, you have set this huge goal of taking on one of the toughest endurance races on the planet, and you've told your family and friends you are going to do it so you don't want to experience fear or embarrassment of failure. On the other hand you realize that certain things are out of your control such as the weather so you try to prepare yourself for any possible situation that might present itself on race day. Control what you can by making better choices and leave the rest up to fate.

Being selfish is a quality most controlling personalities possess and they operate from a place of very high ego. They only consider their own needs. I don't believe it starts out as a mean spirited trait but if you're not careful, your selfish nature can consume you and every ounce of your disposable energy.

When you expend all of your positive energy in pursuit of your dreams at the expense of others, what you're left with is a lot of negative energy and impatience for those around you. In triathlon circles, this is known as over-training.

Over-training can be both physical and mental. On the physical side, over-training leads to temporary injury but on the mental side, you run the risk of being mentally unprepared on race day or conduct yourself in such a way that you offend people for life. Even the professional athletes will admit to being selfish with their time and energy but for them, this is their career. They are training to be in the top 1 percent of the top 1 percent. If you're like me and you simply want to live heart healthy and have really cool experiences in life, a heavy dose of perspective is needed at some point so that selfishness doesn't lead you to burn too many bridges.

Mean, nasty, cranky old bugger! These were the adjectives my wife was using to describe me, especially when I was butting heads with my kids. I have always believed that true leaders lead by example so in my attempt to be a good role model for them health wise, I was succeeding at showing my kids how to live an obsessively selfish life-style.

I had been volunteering as an assistant coach in my son's high school rowing program for his entire high school career. Most of the coaches in our program were formerly part of Canada's National Rowing Program and they were blessed with plenty of international training and race experience. I did not have their same skill level and I knew it. My son loved rowing and gave up playing hockey to row. We traded the hockey dream of playing in the NHL for the dream of a Schoolboy National Championship in rowing and then off to row for school and country.

I want to point out the word "*we*" in that last sentence. Every father I know whose son plays hockey in Canada secretly wants them to be good enough to make it to the NHL. Most hockey parents will never admit to it but you always want to see your kids excel more than you did and if they only took the time to listen to all of your wonderful advice, maybe they would have had half a chance. If you're starting to see how selfish and ridiculous this behavior is, then you stand a chance of turning out OK after all.

I thought I was a great dad, and for the most part I believed that this was true. However, my selfish behavior meant that my son rarely lived up to my performance expectations, and the older he grew, the more we started to argue with each other. We went from unrealistic expectations in hockey to unrealistic expectations in rowing.

My role as the rowing program's conditioning coach put me side by side with the male athletes and I was determined to lead by example and train harder than any of them. I was setting the bar that I expected each of them to surpass. I never stopped to ask Warren what he really wanted. I just selfishly thought that I knew what was best.

In Warren's senior year of high school, I resigned from my coaching duties but ultimately came back into the fold to coach another crew. Warren and I were simply arguing and fighting too much. With a new coach, he went on to have what I will remember as his best rowing season ever. I was fortunate enough to be standing on the dock when he came off the water from his final workout before the finals of the Canadian Schoolboy Regatta. I was there to witness the raw emotion on his face as he realized this was the end of a long chapter for him. This was a treasured moment that I will always have and it may never have happened if I had continued with my selfish ways and continued to push him too hard. As a dad, I finally realized that this was not about me, it was his life to live.

Being selfish is part of the full-distance triathlon experience the first time around, but it doesn't have to continue to be that way if you are smart enough to pay attention and learn from your mistakes. It took about a year after completing my first full-distance triathlon to realize what I had become, to understand that I still hadn't found what I was looking for and to begin the process of trying to understanding why.

I am a student of sport and so long as we are alive we can continue to learn. I love to analyze the professionals and watch championship games because I do believe success leaves clues. I have a playlist of triathlon videos that I watch when I am doing my indoor workouts and many of them are the professionals offering tips on how to be better. You could say that this training technique is where I first realized that repetition perfects performance. You might also think that I am on the lookout for training tips to get faster and while that is partially true, I am also drawn to these videos because of all of the happy smiling faces and I have to ask myself, "why are these people so darned happy?"

Most professional triathletes are earning just enough money to survive. The top 1 percent of the top 1 percent makes it both professionally and financially but everyone else does the sport because they simply love it. Triathlon is an honest sport. If you're really paying attention, it will reveal probably more than you care to know about the person you really are.

My pursuit of finishing the full-distance triathlon revealed to me that anything is possible and if you pay close attention, your journey will reveal to you clues that will ultimately make you a better person.

I am getting better as I grow older. They say that knowing you have a problem is half the problem. I did have a problem. I was selfish, mean, nasty and controlling. Although none of these things were written down as goals on my annual training plan, I was excelling at each and every one of them.

How do we gain new perspective in our lives, in order to become less self-focussed? By listening. Listening is the one skill that I believe we can all improve on. I used to always get a laugh when a certain comedian would say "my wife says I don't pay attention to her or something like that, I don't know I wasn't listening." It's a funny punch line for sure, but not really. I think that too many of us have stopped listening and paying attention to those around us and that is where we start losing our perspective.

What is the real price we pay for selfish behavior? Sometimes it leads to bad choices. In many cases it could mean the destruction of a relationship or the breakup of a family. I sincerely hope that never happens to you. I have been selfish without realizing it for many years. I lost the friendship of two close friends in my forties who I chose to partner with in business. I chose to ignore one of the golden rules of business which is never to do business with friends or family.

In the end, I wasn't dishonest or deceitful; it was simply my selfish and controlling tendencies that left little room for error and expectations that no one could live up to. Very few people could achieve the standards I had set and that included me.

I lived through my thirties doing the best I could for my family. I was running a floundering Promotional Marketing Business

while working at an automotive parts factory. The shift work almost killed me both mentally and physically. It was a real shot to my ego, or so I believed, to take a job that I felt was beneath me. I was suffering from the "Do you know who I am?" complex.
.

I should have just been happy to have a good paying job with benefits and a pension for my family. Looking back, the job itself was not so bad and neither were most of the people. I was able to gain a new appreciation for what factory workers do, and because many of my friends still work in factories today, I can carry on a conversation with them that is both respectful and understanding because of my past experience.

I chose to leave my factory job after seven years. My business was growing, I had paid off my mortgage and there were guys getting laid off who had families to support, so it just felt like the right thing to do. I was making room for someone else in greater need: this is how I sold it to my wife. Maybe I was being selfish in retiring from the factory at forty, but I had convinced myself I was choosing to do the right thing for the greater good. Eventually, the factory closed two years later and I like to think that my stepping aside helped someone else. The irony is that now I coach those same people I used to work with to help them make better choices given what life or fate has presented to them and they have respect for my opinions because I have walked a mile in their shoes.

Here is what selfish people do. They stop listening to reason and they act on emotion directed from self-preservation. I quit a well-paid steady job with benefits in an effort to feed my ego and that was selfish behavior from my family's point of view.

As you can plainly see, selfishness caused many issues for me and I was fully responsible for the mess I had created. It's no wonder I wasn't very happy. I must have upset so many people without even realizing it due to my arrogance.

Looking back now, my wife Robin and my kids are the best things that ever happened to me. They have stood by me while I have tried to figure out what my greater purpose in life is supposed to be. Just last week while I was waiting to pitch this book idea to the producers of a well know reality business TV show, I was texting my son at university and while I was having a difficult time explaining my mid-life crisis book idea to him, his response was "you miss 100 percent of the shots you never take." Now I know these are not his words and I think I first saw them on an inspirational poster back in the 80s, but it's scary how much your kids actually learn from you. Just when you think they are never going to pay attention, they sit there like sneaky little sponges and absorb every word you say.

I want my kids to have the benefit of learning from my mistakes but if I try to be too selfish and control their every move, they won't have the experience of making mistakes to learn from. Learning to get back up and dust yourself off is something we shouldn't try to protect our kids from.

Let's put this into some perspective though. My daughter in grade 9 was asked to the prom by a senior in grade 12. This is not the type of learning experience I am willing to let her have. Mom and dad get to step in and say NO! He is too old. End of conversation. I think that is just good parenting. You may disagree and if so, we agree to disagree. When my teenage daughter is with her own peers, who are her own age and at her own maturity level, she is free to make her own choices and mistakes. We hopefully raised her to make good decisions. Throwing her to

the wolves and hoping she comes out un-
scarred is just stupid.

At any given point in our lives we can act
selfishly. Sometimes the consequences can
be severe and life altering and other times it
can go undetected for years. My selfish behavior was the latter. I didn't aspire to be
mean or angry with people, this is just the
person I became because I was trying too
hard chasing unrealistic expectations. To put
it into triathlon terms, my weakest event is
the swim. The harder I tried to go faster in
the water the slower I would go. I break
down in form and technique and create drag
in the water resulting in a less than stellar
performance.

A good friend of mine who is a very fast
swimmer but looks nothing like what you
would expect a great swimmer to look like
reminded me that the first rule of swimming
well is learning to relax in the water. As
soon as you learn to relax and stop fighting
the water, you will go faster. The same holds
true for selfish behavior, the harder you try
to succeed at everyone else's expense, the
more frustrated you become with less than
perfect results.

I have a wonderful relationship with my bank. I am their customer but we work together. People who like you make it easier to do business with them. The main receptionists name is Betty. I learned her name on day one and over the years, as managers come and go, Betty remains a constant figure at the bank. I look for and say hello to her every time I go to the bank and I know that when the bank doors close for the day and the employees talk about the crazy customers they had to deal with that day, I know that Betty will always have my back. I have no ulterior motive when being respectful and friendly to Betty. But I do understand that if I was selfish and only cared about my own needs and ignored the people around me, no one would care about me and no one would be looking out for me. Acting selfishly is a tough way to go through life.

Beyond Triathlon: Focussing on Relationships

If being positively selfish wasn't going to bring lasting happiness, maybe learning how to be positively selfless would. I know that I am not always selfless and that it is a constant work in progress. Going through the process of becoming a triathlete sharpened my perception to see the value of getting fit: to spend my life on people.

When I crossed the full-distance triathlon finish line and I didn't find that big "lasting happiness" that I was looking for, I could have just as easily moved on to some other new challenge and be done with it. But that wasn't part of the deal. I was on this journey to become a better person and experience life living heart fit and healthy and the sense of emptiness that I was feeling was somehow very wrong. I didn't realize it immediately, but in order to find happiness you have to be attentive to all of the things that you have made second place to reaching your goals. I realized that I needed to serve others by becoming a better husband and father. I needed to find ways to be a better son

and brother, and in all my outside relationships, I would need to become a better listener.

To serve more people, I would have to learn
to be better at being more selfless. What that
means is to put the needs of others before
your own. Now, I'm no Mother Theresa nor
do I pretend to be. Making a conscious effort to be a better listener is a great place to
start. This is how you start to gain more perspective.

One way I became a better listener was for
me to pay closer attention to what other people were saying. We all love the sound of
our own voice and we all want to be heard.
So many times we stop actively listening to
further our own opinion or agenda.

A great way I learned to become an active
listener was to paraphrase what others would
say to me. For example, if my wife said "I
need you to change this light bulb for me," I
could either say "yes dear," because I
wanted to get back to whatever else I was
doing and totally not hear what she was saying, or I could choose to say "OK, which
light bulb do I need to change?" If you paraphrase what people are saying, it engages

your thought process, immediately requiring you to become an active listener.

Actively listening is a sign of respect and that one skill will serve you very well throughout your life. People are happier when you respect them and when people are happy with you, you feel happy in return.

Being a better husband and father or wife and mother can be a little trickier. One way I am trying to be better is by making special time to spend with my wife. For your spouse, a regular date night is the best way to go. I used to plan big surprises around my date nights with my wife. There is a mental dance you can do with the person you love that makes a relationship come alive because they sense that you appreciate them.

There are many stories I could tell but my favorite one was when I was going away to work at a trade show in Toronto, which is an hour's drive from our home. I went to my local shopping mall armed with my credit card and my wife's particular sizes. I went to the mall at 11 a.m. when there would be fewer people shopping and my first stop was to a formal dress store. I walked in and looked the three sales women behind the counter straight in the eyes and I told them that I was taking my wife to a black tie event that evening at the Royal York in Toronto. It was going to be a surprise and I needed their help with everything. Well, let me tell you it was like these women had been sent on a mission from God. They dropped everything and three of them helped me find the perfect dress for my wife. Then I said what's next and they directed me to the lingerie store down the way with permanent smiles and wishing me good luck. I walked into the lingerie store, dress in hand and told the sales women the exact same story and before I knew it I had everything she would need and I was on my way again to the shoe store for my final stop. Once inside the shoe store, again the story was told and the sales people scoured over the many styles to find the perfect shoe to fit the occasion.

I do not enjoy the typical shopping experience. My goal is get in and get out as fast as possible, but this trip, however painful in the pocket book was worth every penny. The sales women at each store loved being able to help me. They were able to play a role in the perfect surprise date. To pull off the perfect surprise for my wife, I simply called home two minutes after leaving the house and asked Robin to check if I had left something on my desk. What she found were three wrapped gift boxes with all of the items I had purchased and a note that read "Meet me at the Royal York on Saturday night in room 516. Your key will be waiting for you at the front desk." My stunned wife called back after about fifteen minutes laughing and said "what's going on?" I just told her to take the kids over to her mom's; it had all been prearranged and meet me at the hotel. There was no black tie event for us to attend that night but we were the stars of the show in the hotel dining room.

I tell you this story to highlight that even a simple date can be turned on its head and be memorable enough to last a lifetime when you take the time to think about your partner's needs first and make them feel appreciated. I like doing special things for my wife because I know I can if I give it a bit of thought, and it makes us both feel very good about choosing to be with each other. How many of you can remember a date night like this with your significant other? To be honest, as I'm writing this, it is reminding me that we are overdue for another adventure. I hope this story will help inspire you to do something special for someone else today. Being selfless will bring you happiness and happiness can be expressed in many great ways.

Being a better father can be a little trickier. Each of us hope that we can teach our kids to have good values and that they will make good decisions on their own. My son and I have had many arguments throughout his teen years and most were instigated by me because I didn't agree with his choices. I was basically teaching my son that arguing and raising your voice was the way to get what you want. I was the alpha male in the home and sometimes I tried to rule with an iron fist. This is not the way to solve your differences. I keep reminding myself that my son chose to go into communications at university and that's a good thing. The world can use more people who are better at communicating with each other.

Much of my stress in my thirties came from feeling like an inadequate provider to my family. We had purchased a brand new home when my wife and I were married and we had the mortgage paid off by the time I turned forty. What could be so wrong with that? Well, looking back I should have felt very proud that my twenty-five year mortgage was paid off in about sixteen years. Once the house was paid off, we purchased a boat and within three months we found ourselves moving to a much bigger and nicer home with a brand new twenty-five year mortgage. I didn't see trouble waiting at the door. With the new home came the new furniture, new landscaping, new lifestyle, new property taxes, etc. We quickly found ourselves living beyond our means at what was essentially the start of the recession. Topped off with the stress of a business deal gone horribly wrong and we had the perfect storm. I have spent the last seven years trying to right the ship and although I have been doing a sufficient job of staying the course, it has taken every ounce of my energy to not have to file for bankruptcy. The only down time I ever experience anymore is when I am sleeping. I strive to achieve more balance, but I'm not giving up.

Being a better dad is about being mentally present for your teenage daughter and making time for her and her friends to do silly things. I don't think I completely embarrass my daughter, and her friends seem to like me. I know this because I can always get them to talk to me when I ask them to spill the beans about Katelyn and the boys who are chasing her at school. I don't tend to stick my head in the sand and I sometimes like to ask awkward questions. After the shock and giggling, 50 percent of the time I get a very interesting answer.

My very good friend Eric who is the father to two teenage daughters has this to say about being there for his daughters and their friends when they need him "You can always call me for a ride if you have been drinking or are in trouble. I won't judge you but I may openly mock you. That is my right as a parent." My friend is a wise man.

Being a better friend simply means being a better friend. It is an ongoing process. Whenever I start to complain around Eric he reminds me that I am no different than anyone else and we all have our own issues to work through.

Humor is usually a quality we look for in friends. If people are funny and fun to be around, then they become good friend material. The closer a person's values are to your own, the better friends you become. It's funny that of all the hockey parents we crossed path with, we haven't remained friends with any of them, but the dance parents who we have known since our daughter was three years old have remained for the most part our best friends. I'm not really sure why that is. I'm not going to say that it's because hockey parents are more competitive than dance parents because I would put money on many dance moms I know in a fight against a hockey parent. Dance moms know how to kick! I think that we have just been blessed to be introduced to a great group of people who have stuck together as a group for many years and we are always looking out for each other. This group puts my needs ahead of their own at times and I try to do the same for them and that makes us all better friends.

Being a better son is a worthy goal. I think many men today who are in their forties and fifties had a similar childhood to mine. Dad went to work, brought home the bacon and left you on your own, hoping you wouldn't get into too much trouble. I remember my dad as an adult always playing sports if he wasn't working. He ran a men's basketball league for years and when I was old enough, I got to play some pick-up with my dad and his friends on a weekly basis for a few years. What I always remember though was the silence in the car on the rides to and from the gym. We had nothing to talk about. The odd time we would discuss something trivial but communication was not our specialty.

My dad is in his seventies now and in failing health. I really have to work hard at warming up to him and finding things to talk about. It's difficult seeing your dad as a shadow of his former self. The way I can be a better son to him is just making the effort to stop in and say hello more often. It seems so simple and yet so difficult at the same time. I have so much on my plate that I simply don't want to make the time and I know I will miss him when he's gone. That's the irony of the situation. I know that when I choose to stop by it makes him happy, even if it is only for a few minutes, so if that is what I need to do to make him happy, then that is what I need to do to be selfless with my dad. We can't change the past, but moving forward, we can all make better choices.

"Find a reason to smile today." In this world we live in, we are constantly bombarded by bad news in the media. Sensationalist bad news sells advertising. I think people crave bad news to justify that their lives aren't so bad after all.

There is something called the law of attraction: surround yourself with enough bad news and you will start to feel bad and inevitably you will only see that bad things are happening. On the flip side, athletes, particularly triathletes tend to be a more positive group of people. Maybe it's the mindset of doing something positive for yourself every day that is ingrained by the training. Maybe it's the fact that other triathletes tend to be positive, happy people. Also, as the law of attraction states, acting positive and happy attracts more of those kinds of people into your life.

I haven't been walking around with a Grinch- like scowl on my face every day. It's just that when you're lucky enough to live long enough to have a midlife crisis, you start asking yourself questions like, "Do I really have to hit my head against the wall every day? Just because everyone else earns a living the traditional way, does that mean I have to as well?" This is the law of attraction at work. Do what you've always done and get what you've always got. The mindset of a triathlete is one of always pushing boundaries to experience life a little different every day. Much like an entrepreneur who works with a blank canvas and creates opportunity every day, a triathlete asks himself, "who am I going to be today?" and then sets out to challenge himself to find the answer.

Four Life Principles Every Triathlete Knows

We can all use more perspective to make better decisions every day.

Most of my thirties were spent chasing hopes and dreams and a career that never materialized the way I envisioned it would. My perspective was always standing on the outside of a bubble looking in. I had no idea what it was going to take to get into that inner circle and I had no idea what I would find once I got there. All I knew and believed is that I wasn't where I was meant to be. I think that when we are in our thirties, we start to settle down and build strong roots for our family. We develop our social status in our community and we get comfortable.

We try to project who we want to be and not who we really are. Maybe this is where people lose perspective. The concept of being "who you want to be" can be confused with "what you want to be" when you try to keep up with the Joneses.

People can lose focus on what is really important in life and they sometimes lose their

way when they get caught up in living beyond their means. Focus shifts from the indi-
viduals needs to a growing family's needs. If
you are lucky enough to have children, they
can consume every last minute of your time,
energy, and sometimes even money you
don't have.

There is nothing wrong with living the
dream and providing for your family, until
you stop to realize that living on borrowed
credit leads to making choices that can haunt
you for years. Your forties is a good time for
reflection.

Bad financial decisions in your twenties and
thirties can lead to a great deal of unwanted
stress. You need to make better choices in
your forties if you want to learn to deal with
that stress and be healthy enough and live
long enough to meet and experience a rich
life with your grandkids. I have a dream of
doing triathlons with my grandkids. I expect
that is a good twenty to thirty years away
and that would plant me firmly into my seventies, and that will be awesome. Between
now and then, I have to be the person every
day who I want people to remember me for
being. The following are four life principles
that were ingrained in me at an early age and
reinforced by my triathlon experiences.

Respect for others regardless of their outward appearance was the first lesson I learned as a triathlete. Respect was actually the key value my parents taught me to have, so for that, I say to them, "thank you."

Triathlon is not just a young person's sport. Triathlon is a sport for every age group and every ability level. To see men and women competing at these distances well into their seventies and eighties is nothing short of inspiring.

My father was the first person to teach me about respect. Respect is simply something that you earn through your actions and deeds. Respect isn't a word that you just toss around. I was brought up to respect my elders, but we do not have to put conditions of age with the giving of respect. I think everyone deserves the benefit of the doubt, and yet they still have to earn our respect. Age alone does not warrant respect. It is your character that either commands a person's respect or pity. When it comes to choosing how you will live your life, healthy or not, your outcome later in life is normally a direct result of your daily decision making process. You didn't become the person you are in one day, one month, or one year. Your reality today is a result of a lifetime of either good or bad decisions compounding over time.

Character is defined as the way someone thinks, feels and behaves. Thinking about a situation gives you perspective. How you feel about the potential outcome of the decisions you make will ultimately cause you to behave one way or the other. If you think, feel and behave in a way that leads others to believe that your life is a precious gift, and that you truly value it, then of course you will have their respect.

The alternative is to live your life as you please, aware and yet unmoved by the obvious consequences, always in denial, reasoning that you are no worse than anyone else. Living your life no worse than anyone else is the way most people go through life and if you are reading this book, maybe it's that very thought process that has led you to think and feel that it is time for a change. You see, the great thing about a person's character is that we all have greatness within us. Once you decide that enough is enough and you want to make a change, people will respect and accept you for who you are today. When I say that respect has to be earned, be aware that the road ahead is going to be tough. There will be days that you want to give up and quit, but the kind of character that commands respect is evident in your decision to continue to invest in yourself every day. The question you need to ask yourself is who are you going to be today? If you are overweight, that is what you are. If you are working hard every day to solve that problem, who you are is a person on a mission. Make that distinction and people will respect that. Live your day with self-confidence and pride and that will define who you are, not what you were. The only decision left to make is to go out and do the same thing again tomorrow.

I love being an age group triathlete because triathletes understand that we all have greatness within us and that winners don't always come in first place. The first and only goal of every triathlete who steps up to the starting line is to finish. Being brave enough to say "I can" and then following those words up with action shows a person's true character. Certain actions command respect. Others, most assuredly do not.

In fairness, every generation on this planet grows a little wiser than the generation before, and my parents and their parents did not have the same understanding of our bodies nor the resources to educate themselves the way we do today. However, when it comes to giving respect to people of my generation and my kids' generation based on how they live their lives, I tend to get a little more cynical.

I can't believe that with everything we know about smoking today that kids and adults still continue to smoke. It just blows my mind when I go to local high school to coach rowing and pass the smoking pits. What a sight it is to see a group of fifteen year-old boys and girls smoking and spitting continuously because they can't stand the taste in their own mouths. How is it that these youth do not respect their own health and well-being? Some might argue that these kids are just trying to fit in, but as adults of good character, we need to look for opportunities to mentor and coach young people who are falling through the cracks in life. If you are a person of good character, then you have something to offer. It takes time to build relationships and to be a good role model, but in the end, you cannot underestimate the potential of your actions if you decided to become important in the life of a child, even if that child is not your own.

Six years ago, I met a young boy named Ian who has earned my respect. Ian was just starting high school, in grade 9 at the time. He had come out to one of our first rowing practices and all I can remember thinking at the time from my first impression was, "how was this scrawny little kid possibly going to row?" I judged him before I even gave him a chance. My understanding was that school was a challenge for him and he was considered an "at risk" student. Not a great first impression, but Ian kept coming out every day to every practice and as it turns out, Ian wanted to be a coxie, but he also wanted to work out with the rowers to build up a little muscle strength. The simple fact that he was reliable and wanted to make an investment in his health every day was enough to earn my respect, but there was an underlying opportunity to do a little more.

Over the four years I had the pleasure of coaching Ian, rowing became his passion, and I believe from talking with his parents that being a valued member of the rowing crew helped keep him on track in school. Ian and I learned a lot from each other, but one of the most basic traits I wanted to teach him was about character and respect. His parents were fantastic people and I'm sure he got his great work ethic from home. The opportunity to teach young people about character and respect is a responsibility we all share. I always told my crews that respect was not something that was automatically given to you because of who you thought you were, it was given to you only because you had the character to deserve it. A great tradition of our St. Catharines Rowing Club is that when any club crew wins a medal, upon leaving the medal podium, the medal gets tucked into your shirt. Gloating or boasting are not qualities that are supported or encouraged. This is a great example of both character and respect for fellow athletes.

I firmly believe that *the true character of a person can be measured by what you do when nobody is watching you.* When you conduct yourself with good character, you will earn the respect of others. With Ian under my wing, I wanted to demonstrate how leaders lead by example and how to earn the respect of others by making the right impression.

Henley Island in St. Catharines, Ontario is a world- famous rowing course, and fortunately for me it is my home course. One-time use plastic water bottles are one of the biggest challenges we face on Henley Island. Why? Because apparently one of the things many parents can't seem to teach their kids is that when you are finished with garbage, your garbage goes in the garbage can.

Despite carefully placed and highly visible garbage cans all over the Island, kids just can't seem to grab the concept that empty plastic water bottles go in the garbage can. I simply don't get it. It's not that complicated, and yet every day, there are at least 100 new water bottles strewn all over the island. So rather than complain about it and point fingers, I simply walk around and pick them all up as I go about my business. Most of the kids just stand and watch or ignore what I am doing altogether. They don't get it. To these kids, I'm just another parent picking up their mess after them. All it would take is for one person to follow my lead, then another to follow them, and a cultural shift in respect could happen. *In a triathlon, the consequence for getting caught littering on the racecourse is immediate disqualification.* We are guests in the community and if we want the communities support and respect for years to come, we have to continually earn it.

I explained to Ian and all of my crew that people are always watching. Some might even be quietly paying attention. The club captain has taken notice, and when he sees our crew cleaning up every day, he has more respect for our crews, our coaches and our school. You never know when good karma will come back to repay you. I choose to do the right thing because I want to earn peoples' respect and you never know who you might influence in the process. I choose to do the right thing because it makes me feel better as a person, so even when no one is watching, if you have character, you will choose to do the right thing. Ian joined me many days cleaning up the boathouse and Island grounds because he knew I wasn't asking him to do anything that I wasn't prepared to do myself. In my mind, that is mutual respect. I look forward to teaching that lesson all over again to the junior girls I will be coaching this season.

When it comes to triathlon, I know how hard I have to train. It comes down to spending hundreds of hours on your own swimming, biking, and running. The only one who can see you is the only person you are competing with and that is yourself. No one is watching me train, so I can go as easy or as hard as I like. Because I know what is required to get to the finish line, I assume that everyone who registers for the race has gone through the same training that I have. I know how difficult it can be and the sacrifices that must be made in order to put the hours in to successfully complete the race. For that reason alone, everyone who is brave enough to say "I CAN" and attempt this race shares a mutual respect for each other.

The best thing about the people who compete at the full triathlon distance level is the mutual respect that both the pros and the age groupers have for each other. You won't find this kind of mutual admiration in any other sport and you will often hear the pros saying it's the age groupers that inspire them, not the other way around.

As age group athletes, we respect the pro's talent and they respect our iron will to complete the race. This is the only sport that I can think of where the pros compete on the same playing field as the amateurs and where you will find more people coming back to the finish line to support and cheer in athletes who take the full seventeen hours to complete the race. That, my friend, is mutual respect for your fellow competitor. One of the best traditions at every full-distance triathlon race is that the winning profession-als come back at midnight to present the fin-isher medals to the final competitors who cross the finish line at the official end of the race. The finish at midnight is quite the party. You're happy you made it to the fin-ish line and that you didn't die in the process and so are 5000 cheering spectators. They will cheer you in by name and it is one of the most amazing experiences you can have in life. In that one moment in time, you have earned the respect of 5000 complete strangers, not because of what you did while they were watching you cross the finish line, but because of what you did for the past sev-enteen hours and all of the months of train-ing it took to get you there when they couldn't see you.

Acceptance. When it comes to long distance triathlon, if you are brave enough to say, "I can do this" and step up to the starting line, you are immediately accepted by your fel-low competitors regardless of any visible disabilities. You should never judge a book by its cover and you need only watch any triathlon World Championship video on the internet to see that we are only limited by our own presumptions and biases.

I was reminded earlier this fall when I moved my swim training indoors that I should never judge people on appearances alone. When you go to the pool to do lane swimming, you try to seed yourself with other swimmers of your own speed and ability so that you can push each other and not get in each other's way as the workout unfolds.

I had joined the local masters swim program to work with a friend of mine who was running the program. Christine is a distance swimmer and when I first met Christine in the water, she was training to swim across Lake Ontario. In her training, she would swim with a harness attached to her waist pulling a kayak loaded up with her two young daughters. Her daughters would sit in the kayak reading books and eating snacks as mom pulled them up and down the Welland Flat-water Swim Course. If anyone could help me swim faster it would be Christine.

Upon arriving for my first workout, I noticed a woman making her way to the pool deck on crutches, and having competed with Para-athletes in other races, this should not have fazed me one bit. I'm not sure why I was thinking the way I was, but I remember wanting to make sure I got into a different lane than her because I didn't want to be stuck behind her, compromising my own workout.

I was introduced to Martha and we shook hands, exchanged pleasantries and then started our respective warm up laps. Martha was missing one of her legs from the knee down and while my assumption was that she would be slower due to this "handicap" all I can remember seeing was her passing by with ease in the lane next to me.

I should have known better. After all, I have been a triathlete now for over four years, and if long distance triathlons have taught me anything, it is that if you believe in yourself you can accomplish anything.

In general, I think that I am quite accepting of other people and even more so if they are making an attempt to better themselves. It takes a lot of courage to join into an endurance race with a physical disability, whether it is obvious or not. When I see other athletes who are assuredly many pounds heavier than I am, it's hard not to be able to draw on that inspiration when your day starts to get a little tough. I know how hard the race can be for me given the heat, humidity, and other environmental factors that make up the difficulty of a full-distance triathlon race. If someone with greater challenges than me can do it, what do I have the right to complain about?

Full-distance finishers will tell you that the race is more mental than it is physical and that is the million dollar secret to succeeding every day. Challenging yourself to finish a full-distance triathlon race is an opportunity to see what you are made of on that given day. It is the ultimate test of both physical and mental strength. Unlike other sports where there are clear winners and losers, the first and only goal of the day is to get to the finish line and everyone who finishes the race is accepted as a winner in the same way that the actual time winners of the race are. This community of support and acceptance plays an enormous role in an athlete's ability to finish such a grueling race.

Finishing a full-distance triathlon puts you into an exclusive club of very exceptional and accepting members. People don't care what position you placed, they simply want to celebrate that you shared a common goal and you experienced it together. We are all equal as athletes when we are brave enough to choose to step up to that line.

Balance. Too much of anything is never a good thing. If you train too much, ignoring the needs of those around you, you risk alienating them forever. Train too much, ignoring your own need for rest, and you risk damaging your body in other ways. Deprive yourself of the foods you love and you will learn to hate the process of exercise and living healthier altogether.

I like to look at balance as the great equalizer. Balance and perspective go hand in hand. Having perspective allows you to bring more balance into your life. Each and every one of us should have enough time in the day to invest forty-five to sixty minutes on your heart health. Presuming you sleep seven hours a day, that leaves you with sixteen hours to get done everything you need to do in a day. What you do with that sixteen hours comes down to your own decision making process. It sounds simple enough because it is. We spend way too much of our available time serving other peoples' agendas or sitting watching screens. Perspective helps you to manage your time better. For example, if you go to bed by 11 p.m. most nights, you can wake up at 6 a.m. to work out for an hour and by 7 a.m. you have that investment in the bank and you are ready to tackle your day. That is simply one of many

choices you can choose to make. Some decisions bring you closer to your goals while
others take you further away. If you live
your life with balance, there is always time
for the things that are important to you, like
finding the time to relax on the couch with
someone you love. Whatever it is that is important to you in your life, you need to have
balance so that you don't let any part of it
slip away. Spending too much time on any
one thing will lead to imbalance and a lonely
difficult existence.

We will cover balanced eating in the chapter
"Eating Well Makes You Feel Good." What
I would like to talk about here is balance as
a philosophy for healthy living.

You have to think of your life as a three-
sided pyramid: Body, mind and spirit. If you
neglect to maintain any one of the three
walls, the structure will collapse. The concept of body, mind and spirit working in
harmony has been around for centuries.
Here's a summary of my best days on this
planet.

When I train in the morning, I feed my body
with the exercise it needs to maintain a
healthy internal system. We all know that

exercise is the most proactive, preventative thing we can do for our health. When we exercise, our body releases endorphins into our brains that help us to be more energetic, alert and better problem solvers in general. Spirit for me represents your conscience. With a guilt- free conscience, strong body and healthy mind, you can accomplish anything.

Of the three internal systems, I struggle with my mind the most. Working out is the easy part. I have been at it now for over seven years and my body rarely fights back with any aches and pains. I know that I always feel great after a workout and I reward myself both physically and mentally with a glass of chocolate milk. You would think that chocolate milk with all of that sugar would be on the no-eat list but when consumed at the right time and for the right reasons, many things that society paints as bad for us may also serve a useful purpose. Just as drinking flat soda on the racecourse fuels my body's immediate sugar needs, chocolate milk helps to rebuild my body after my workout. Because I am drinking it intentionally, for a purpose, it is the balanced choice for that time. After your workout is over, your body has produced endorphins and that has your brain firing on all cylinders. Unfortunately, the effect is just temporary. I often joke with people saying that if you work out in the evening, all of your best thinking will be wasted while you are sleeping but you will have the most incredible dreams.

So how do you set out to have a guilt- free conscience, to have a quiet spirit? For me, a guilt- free conscience comes from doing your best to do right by others every day. Most of us are taught the difference between right and wrong from a very young age. When I say most of us, I am fully aware that there are many kids today who have been and are being raised without this basic common knowledge. I really like the concept that it takes a village to raise a child because with the right amount of patience, care and compassion, I believe that kids are smart enough to see the difference between right and wrong by the example we choose to set for them. We lead by example, and in turn do ourselves the kindness of bringing peace to our environment.

Purpose is probably the most misunderstood word ever to be tossed around in the fitness industry. Ask ten different fitness "experts" from club members, to trainers, to club owners, to health and wellness consultants and I guarantee you will get ten completely different answers. Everyone is going to have a different definition of purpose to support their program.

What I am going to ask of you is to use a little common sense when choosing your fitness activities. Try to see the business behind the business of the fitness industry for just a minute and ask yourself, "what do I really need to do to live a heart healthy existence, and what does that even mean?"

My wife goes to boot camps and she spins at our studio. Boot camp beats her up and makes her sore for days. She says things like "I'm really sore today because we did 100 burpees yesterday." When I ask what the purpose of that workout was and how does it fit into her workouts for the rest of the week she just gets mad at me and says not everyone is training to be a triathlete. My usual response is that you don't have to be a triathlete to train like one. You just have to train with purpose. That just makes sense. Beating yourself up with no rhyme or reason doesn't make sense to me. I'm in pretty good shape and I don't beat myself up, even when I cross train with weights because I do it at the right times and with a progressive purpose. I have a plan to get stronger and a plan to rest. Foundationally, I have an annual plan.

My annual plan is very simple: choose to do something good for your heart every day and train in a manner that the activities don't change, only the time or distance spent doing them either increases with volume to build endurance or decreases allowing for rest. I never stop. I simply adjust the volume according to my plan. A triathlete trains twelve months a year. We start with our big race day and work eight months back from that date. This is when our sport- specific training starts. The other four months are spent on recovery, maintenance and cross training for variety. We do other activities that keep our aerobic endurance strong without burning out on the sport we love. I add in hockey and erg workouts during this time to keep my mind fresh. For a hockey player, aerobic endurance reduces the amount of time you need to recover from a shift. When I skate hard and come off of the ice, my heart rate is fully recovered after about thirty seconds, while my friends continue to suck wind for minutes.

For me, living a HeartFit life has meant reducing my risk factor for diseases that can be caused or exacerbated by a sedentary lifestyle. Like you, I want to feel young in body and mind for as long as I possibly can. Having a strong healthy body and mind affords me the opportunity to feel young enough to enjoy my kids in an active way.

Taking it one step further, I see people in their seventies and eighties today who are as healthy as I am and living the life I just described because they have positive perspective and good balance in life.

Many professional athletes, most who were at the top of their game in their twenties, go on to lead an unhealthy life after retirement. Typically, the triangle of body, mind and spirit shifts out of balance. This can be a result of any excess that they allow to overtake them. Money won't fix the problems this will create, and wealth is not the answer to lasting health and happiness. I don't want the best doctors money can buy. In fact, I don't want to have to rely on any doctors at all.

I have been saying for the past four years that you don't have to be a triathlete to learn

from one. Because it takes years of training
and specifically six to eight months of event
specific training to complete a full-distance
race, every workout a triathlete does serves a
specific purpose. You have to have balance
in your life to train that long for a one day
event and not get the triangle out of whack.

There is an annual cycle that a triathlete follows that allows us to prepare our bodies for
race day. We begin by strengthening our
bodies in the off season with weight training
when our muscles have plenty of time to recover. This is called periodized training.
Then we shift into base and build months
where we do sport specific training and sys-
tematically increase our body's ability to
cope with the added stress that will be
placed on us from an endurance perspective.
With our twelve month training plan unfold-
ing, every week we follow a simple routine
that includes six days of workouts followed
by one day of rest and recovery.

Your purpose each week is to have days that
build strength and days which build endurance. One of the first things you learn about
triathlon training which you can apply to
your own workouts is that you can't train for
both strength and endurance in the same session and you must allow for adequate rest

between each session. On top of that training plan, you have to have your body peak both physically and mentally on race day or everything you have worked so hard for may come crashing down around you with a DNF (did not finish) result. Now fear might prompt you to say "what if I did all that work and didn't finish?" The good news is that you would still be the fittest you have probably ever been in your life and your quality of life will have improved dramatically. I don't see the down side to reaching that point of fitness.

You may have realized by now that the race itself isn't the endurance part of the sport, it's the commitment to the journey which takes years of training that offers the greatest endurance challenge. What I can tell you is that as a former fat guy at forty, I have been training now with purpose for seven years and I have been relatively injury free. I am never sore anymore from training. Your body might get fatigued at times, but the next day you will be ready to go at it again. All you likely need is a little more sleep.

For my last race in Mexico, my wife and I purposely chose to stay at an all-inclusive resort in Mexico. It wasn't near the start of the race like I would normally like but it was the right choice for my family. The race isn't just about me. I had to make sure my fans were getting the race experience they deserved as well. While I was out in the hot sun doing my thing, my family and friends were swimming in the hotel pool drinking margaritas, and I was happy for them. My family's spectator experience in Louisville was not so pleasant and I wanted everyone to win this time around. After an amazing day of triathlon racing, we all joined together for the post-race victory celebration. The party was awesome and you've got to love a life built around purpose, balance and passion.

The Entrepreneurial Spirit-
The Way of the Triathlete

Entrepreneurs make up a substantial amount of the new workplace environment and these people typically don't have deep pockets and the odds are not on their side for success. This is not a formula for happiness but every now and then another entrepreneur makes it big and that fuels the fire of optimism for the rest of us. I guess you can say that real entrepreneurs don't fear the outcome because they understand that there will be some pain during the process.

A triathlete who is new to the sport looks at other triathletes and they see that most settle in at the shorter race distances. They test the waters before making any real commitments, much like a first time entrepreneur who doesn't give up their day job before jumping in with both feet. Every now and then however, one or two of their new triathlete friends will decide to take the leap of faith and tackle the full-distance triathlon. Some will face the challenge head on and survive the training and race day, others will stumble and fall and not be so successful. Whether you get to cross the finish line or not, you inevitably learn something about yourself, something you didn't already know. You get to see how hard you can get hit in life and how strong your resolve is to get back up and keep on going.

As an entrepreneur in my professional life, you can start to see what attracts me to triathlon in my personal life. It's all about the pursuit of excellence and deciding that I want more from my life than just punching a clock and collecting a wage. Arnold Schwarzenegger said, "Ask not what you want to be but who you want to be."

I ran an introduction to triathlon and spinning program at the high school level for one year and the teachers all said the same thing, they would like to teach the kids one thing but the curriculum demanded that they teach something else. They wanted to be teachers, but they didn't know how to become the teacher who they most wanted to be, "themselves" and by being themselves, they would feel as though that had the freedom to make a difference.

Trying to keep up with the Joneses and meet other people's expectations is not a formula for success or happiness and it is operating from a place of very high ego. If a beginner

triathlete tried to keep up with an elite triathlete, they would need to spend tens of thousands of dollars on equipment and training
without having put in any of the base training, years of pain, suffering and striving for
improvement that got the elite athlete to
where they are today. There are no shortcuts
in life and fitness. You get rewarded for
paying a price and that price is years of hard
work and dedication.

In my mind, success is having the freedom
to do what makes you feel happy every day.
I do have entrepreneur friends who are very
successful and they are no different from me
so that knowledge gives me hope. I have one
friend in particular that is almost too successful and with that level of success comes
challenges that I'm sure has him losing
sleep. So what does he do to relieve
stress? He bought a bike and sometimes, on
rare occasions, such as when I come to visit,
he even finds time to ride it.

I have also had the privilege to meet many
professional triathletes who are no different
from I am other than age, and they also inspire me and motivate me to keep moving
forward. Again balance is the key. Understanding that life, health, and happiness are
all part of conscious decisions that we get to

make every day is what inspires me. Understanding that there is a price to be paid and
that usually involves hard work is what triathlon has taught me about myself. Triathlon
has taught me that I am stronger both mentally and physically than I ever thought I
could be.

In triathlon training, at the start of every new
12 month season, we write down our season
goals. Then we write down our "limiters." Limiters are the things that we need to
improve about ourselves to have the desired
outcome we want to have on race day. We
don't stop training the things we are good at
just because we are already good at it. We
keep striving to get better at what we already
know and then we make special time to
work on the things that need improvement.

When you apply this mindset to your life
and your career, it forces you to ask yourself
some pretty tough questions. It doesn't matter what you do to earn a living, if you're
not constantly improving your knowledge
and skill sets to stay ahead of the learning
curve, you're falling behind. If you're ignoring an area that definitely needs improvement, you're falling behind. In triathlon,
your first and only goal of the day is to make
it to the finish line, but once you gain more

experience and confidence, your belief system starts to change as does your expectations for what is really possible.

If you are feeling depressed right now, please know that my story is not meant to depress you. It's my way of letting you know that I have shared your struggle, I have gained a fresh new perspective and I have found solutions for my life that work. I live most days being the person *who I want to be*. I attract other successful people into my life who believe in me and add value to our shared experiences. Together we are creating a movement that is making a difference. We are becoming important in peoples' lives.

Happiness and success are not always measured by money. In the past, I often found myself asking my family why they were never happy and I finally realized that they were simply giving back to me what I was giving to them. It was the law of attraction. I was outwardly projecting unhappiness and they were giving it back to me in spades. Try smiling at someone for no particular reason and watch them smile back at you. Happiness is infectious and it's what inspires me most days. Smiling is free. It is a selfless act that brings happiness and success into your world.

Earlier in my career while I was still in College, I was working for the St. Catharines Blue Jays who were the single A farm club for the Toronto Blue Jays Baseball Club. My boss Rick was the general manager of the club. Rick would become one of the very few people whom I would later consider to be one of my most influential mentors. Rick was always smiling. It didn't matter how much was hitting the fan, he always smiled and tried to solve the problem. Smiling was his way of diffusing difficult situations and getting everyone to calm down and sort through problems logically.

One day I was asked to drive to the Buffalo airport in the new community club van to pick up MLB player Fred McGriff from the airport. I excitedly said yes and off I went. When I got to the Buffalo airport, the road was one way, and three lanes across in front of the terminal. Normally when you parallel park you are doing it on the right side of the vehicle and I am very used to parallel parking. In Buffalo, because of the one-way traffic, I could also park on the left side of the road in the metered parking spots. Not being used to parallel parking on the left side, I opened the driver's side door to get a better look at the curb when "BANG", the door crunched right into the parking meter! This was not my best moment. Neither was the idea of taking a pair of vice grips to the door to try to un-crumple the damage.

When I got back to the office, I had no choice but to show Rick what I had done. With his usual smile, he surveyed the damage and just said we'd fix it. I knew he was angry but he never made me feel small or useless. What point would that have served other than to make Rick feel good to vent in an obviously frustrating situation. Rick used the law of attraction to get the outcome he wanted, an honest employee that accepted responsibility for his mistakes and a harmonious platform to move forward.

Triathlon is one of the fastest growing sports among adults between 35 and 55 all over the world. Why? I believe that the law of attraction has a lot to do with it. People of this age start looking at their lives with new perspective and they seriously consider to how they can make improvements in their life without diminishing the quality of the experiences they enjoy. One of the fastest growing trends in full-distance triathlons is the concept of

corporate challenges where business execu-
tives join training groups to build their social and professional networks, using the
law of attraction to meet like- minded people and grow together.

In my search for lasting happiness, I thought
that by doing one monumental thing like
crossing the full-distance triathlon finish line
would provide the shining light and wisdom
that I was searching for sent straight down
from the heavens. Yes, I have been called an
idiot on more than one occasion so you are
not alone in thinking it too. They say that the
full triathlon distance race is more about the
journey than it is about the destination. I
never really considered my life to be a journey, more of a rambling through time trying
to hold everything together with duct tape.
My father-in-law should get a kick out of
this, as he holds everything you can't nail
down together with duct tape.

Completing the full-distance triathlon gives
you a sense of pride knowing you explored
your limits and you survived. However, limits are just perceptions and not really limits
at all. Today I am fitter and wiser than I was
on my first full-distance attempt so my limits have changed. I expected more from my-

self in my second attempt in both race results and training effort. When I was training
the first time around I was unhappy and un-
sure. Today I am both happy and optimistic
that everyone is in this journey together with
me.

Since my first full-distance race, I have de-
veloped a training program for high school
students where I bring thirty spin bikes into
the school for a week and teach kids the basics of spinning, triathlon, and motivation. I
have learned quite a bit about my body and
how it works and reacts to specific exercise
and nutrition and I love sharing that
knowledge with students. By the time the
week of training is over, I make real connec-
tions with these kids. With the last group, I
let them all know that they would be crossing the finish line in Mexico with me. They
were all in my head at some point during the
race. As I think back to their smiles and con-
versations, I realize that serving others is a
very rewarding experience to cherish in life.

The experiences of triathlon have changed
my life. Success is simply understanding
who you are going to be and choosing to be
that person each and every day. Success can
be as simple as being important in the life of
a child or living every day with the certainty

and knowledge that you have a plan and purpose for your life. No one will think less of
you for deciding to become a better person.

Being Positive

There are really just two types of people: those who say *I can*, and those who say *I can't*. Either way, whichever you believe, you are absolutely right.

To take on the challenge of finishing a full-distance triathlon, you definitely have to believe you can do it. That confidence comes from a progressive belief system. When I turned forty and weighed almost 220 pounds, I knew I was out of shape, but I had been a good high school athlete and I thought my six foot frame hid the weight well. I was kidding myself for a long time into thinking that I was healthy, or at least just as healthy as the next guy. We tend to do that a lot. We compare ourselves with other people our own age to make ourselves feel better.

I used to look at the other guys at the factory when I was in my thirties who were my age or younger who were completely obese and comparing myself to them would make me feel good. I remember thinking, "wow, I don't ever want to be like that guy and I'm not even close, therefore my weight must be reasonably ok. I can drop ten quick pounds if I want to shape up."

Here's the bad news: heart disease, which is the number one killer of adults in North America doesn't care how much you weigh. Sure, extra weight plays a large role in complications leading to heart disease, but many people who are "thin" are equally likely to succumb to this disease if they are not heart healthy. Body shape and image is not a true reflection of heart health. I have many thin friends who are not heart healthy, they are just skinny. I hate it when people call me skinny; I often correct them and say I prefer to be called fit.

I often wondered why it is so difficult for people to really understand what it means to live heart fit. I was at the doctor's office the other day and the receptionist there asked me how my new indoor cycling studio was going. She is a prime candidate for the studio because we specialize in helping people who aren't fit learn the basic steps of becoming heart fit through non-impact exercise. Her response to me about the studio was "I would love to come to your studio but I can't because I have bad knees." I politely smiled and said "that's too bad you feel that way," and ended the conversation.

The reason many people who are overweight have bad knees is because they are over-weight. Spinning and swimming are both non-impact sports that put little to no pressure on your knees while engaged in the sport. These are two activities that people who are overweight should consider in their attempt to reclaim a healthy weight. There is a video on YouTube that I first saw a few years ago about an obese man in his thirties and his desire to run in the Boston Marathon (search - "the most inspiring video you will ever watch" and click on the video of the man running in the red jacket). Over a period of about two years, he started walking, swimming and spinning. He gradually lost the weight and his transformation was simply inspiring. You know he changed his eating habits as well, but it just goes to show that nothing is impossible. It just depends on how bad you want something and if your *Why Factor* is stronger than the excuses you can come up with about having bad or sore knees.

How do you tactfully tell someone who is overweight that the reason their knees hurt is because your body was not designed to carry that much weight in the first place? I think people who are overweight believe that the mountain is just too hard to climb. They fear the process so don't bother to even try.

When I started to train for triathlons, I had already been running for three years so I believed that I could successfully finish a triathlon race. My only concerns and doubts were about finishing the swim. It wasn't because I didn't know yet that I didn't know how to swim, it was because when I was younger, I played baseball at a competitive level and had to retire due to a recurring shoulder injury. When I retired in my twenties, my throwing shoulder was pretty much toast.

I was about forty-three when my shoulder became problematic again. I couldn't sleep on that shoulder at night. The slightest pressure on my left shoulder was like a mild toothache that drives you crazy after twenty minutes or so. My initial thought was that it was the old baseball injury coming back to haunt me. It must be arthritis. That's what happens to old people when they get old, right? Wrong! This was at about the same time that I got in the pool to start my swim training. Without even thinking about it, after only a couple of weeks of swimming, one night I realized the pain was completely gone. I was working the joints and muscles

in my shoulders again through non-impact
exercise and making my shoulders stronger.
The pain was gone and has never returned.
Not a single pill was needed, just some good
old fashioned exercise.

Luckily I didn't think to myself, "I can't
swim, my shoulders could never take it, old
sports injury, you know." Instead I just decided to get myself to the pool and get into
the water and good things started to happen.
The great thing about non-impact sports like
swimming and biking is that they are a great
place to start building a stronger heart if
your joints and muscles can't support your
current weight.

People fear the loss, process, and outcome
of change. They feed their minds with "what
if" statements. What do we risk when we
start something new? We risk failure and
embarrassment and that's why whenever
something new is suggested to us, our natural reaction is to say "I can't" followed by
"what if this happens?"

Let's try a simple experiment. I want you to
ask the next person you see who is not a
small child if they would like to run in a
marathon with you this year and see what
they say. Unless they are a runner, my guess

is their reaction will be something like "I can't do that because…"

When you were a child, one of the first tests in kindergarten you had to pass was learning to tie your shoes. Before anyone ever showed you how, you repeatedly practiced on your own shoes. The task seemed nearly impossible to complete. I was reminded by my son's kindergarten teacher when Velcro straps had replaced shoe laces that she had yet to meet an able bodied adult who was incapable of tying up their shoes.

Your belief system is just your current perspective. Your perspective changes with experience. The more you experience, the more you believe you can do. If you live a life where nothing ever changes, then you believe nothing can change. If you live your life in such a way that you have a clear goal and a path to follow to reach that goal, your perspective and your belief system will change accordingly.

If you had asked me seven years ago if I would ever do a full-distance triathlon and try to qualify for the world championships, I would have said something like, "I can't do that and who in their right mind would even want to try?" It's funny how small steps

forward can change your belief system.
When I was asked that same question before
my race in Cozumel, my answer was "my
time for my last race was just under fourteen
hours. I made some beginner mistakes that
cost me two hours. If I train with interval
work to increase my speed and make fewer
mistakes, I can get down to eleven hours and
at that point, anything can happen." Either
way I know I will have a personal best time.

I approached that same question by saying
"how can I" as opposed to "I can't." That
mental adjustment along with a new and improving belief system made all of the difference in the world.

Some people crave change: they look for the
next great challenge in life. These people
will do the full-distance triathlon race once
and say "been there, done that." They get
their souvenir t-shirt and move on. These are
the people who brag for the rest of their
lives that they were a triathlete. I guess this
is why the purists in the sport don't like the
finishers tattoo, they don't like to brag. They
just want to get better.

I am a purist, but I also like my tattoo. I like
to think that I am an ambassador for the
sport of triathlon. As a forty-eight year old

man, I have a new opinion of what getting old looks like and it looks nothing like Santa Claus. I have some new role models in my world who look like I do now and they are almost twice my age. They may have a few more wrinkles and a little more grey hair but they are living life heart fit and experiencing youthful living because they choose to invest in themselves every day and say "I can." This is the power of positive thinking.

What do challenging experiences teach us about ourselves? They teach us that we are capable of doing more. When I first started running, five kilometres seemed like a very long way. After finishing my first 5k race, I distinctly remember watching and listening to some other runners at the finish line asking each other, "Who wants to go for a run now? That was a good warm up." I remember thinking to myself that these people must be crazy, we just ran five kilometers! The next thing I remember was watching the group of them heading off for their run and it was at that moment that I realized that I could go farther; I just had to change my belief system again.

Going farther and believing in yourself comes from the process of achieving your daily goals. I come from the promotions industry so when I started my journey, I had some t-shirts made that said "Today I Win" I will finish what I started, I will reach my goal. Every night I would lay out my shoes, socks, running shorts and I would fold my shirt on top of the pile so the first thing I saw in the morning was that message.

I didn't really need to lay my clothing out like that but in the beginning, it worked for me. It was the repetition and the emotional trigger that I needed. On the days I didn't feel like getting out of bed to go for a run, I just looked at that shirt and reminded myself of my *Why Factor*. I needed to invest in my heart that day and off I went. I am where I am today because I set realistic and achievable daily goals and I just decided to feel like a winner every day.

Today I use a glow in the dark silicone wrist band that simply reads Heartfit365 PERSPECTIVE – CHOICES – OUTCOME. It's on my wrist 24/7 and it reminds me to make good decisions all day long, 365 days a year.

Having a healthy heart is a process, it is not a destination. Daily fitness is a moving target that is relative to who you are and what your fitness level is at any given point in your life. It is merely a measurement from a window in time.

Crossing the full-distance triathlon finish line for the first time is nothing short of surreal. You experience a huge sense of accomplishment and your belief system goes up a significantly big notch. The thing is that you don't have to be a triathlete to have that sense of accomplishment. I often tell people to go out and sign up for something new and exciting that they never imagined themselves doing before. Find an event or something to reward yourself with for becoming the new fit person you are.

Being fit will definitely make you feel good about yourself, but true happiness comes from something else. Sometimes, as I mentioned earlier, we become obsessed with our goals and become selfish in our behavior. So how do you remain positive and reach your goals without being too selfish? The answer is balance and to have balance, you need to find a way to be better at the relationships that surround you.

Mental Toughness

It's been said that finishing a full-distance triathlon race is more mental than it is physical and that is very true. Henry Ford once said "whether you believe you can or you believe you can't, you're right."

What is it that stops you from getting out of bed every morning and doing something good for your heart? Fear. Fear of loss, process or outcome. We fight daily battles with our minds between taking the right way or the easy way. On average you make 612 decisions every day. 612 choices to either act or do nothing.

For me, being mentally tough is about building on my belief system. The first day I went out to run 5k I believed I could do that distance. I believed that I should be able to do that. Then reality slapped me in the face and knocked me down a notch. I had a choice to make. Do I turn around and go home before anyone sees me looking so foolish or do I take another step forward? I chose to keep moving forward.

I believed that it was possible for me to walk and jog to finish that 5k distance on that day and it was that mental conviction that got me through it. If you had asked me on that day if I believed that one day, maybe when I was forty eight, that I would be competing in full-distance triathlons around the world, I would have said you were crazy because there was no way I believed that was possible.

Your belief system is a fluid thing and it absolutely directs you in life. As with business or in your personal life, if you are not constantly growing, changing and experiencing new things, you are considered to be stagnant or irrelevant. Some might even say that you are stuck living in the past.

I struggled with living in the past. Hung up on my past hopes and dreams choosing to live in the glory days of my mind instead of carving out new adventures for my future. In order to be the person you want to be ten years from now, you need to start being that person today. You don't need to wait for someone else to give you permission to move forward in your life.

We kick the rust off and move forward by challenging ourselves to experience something new. For runners, the 5k race turns into a 10k, then turns into a half marathon, and then a full marathon. As you experience more, you will believe that you can achieve more.

For most full-distance triathletes, there is a certain point in the race that I referred to earlier called "the wall." It can be experienced by both professionals and amateurs alike. It's the point in the race where things aren't going exactly according to plan and your mind starts building a case for some much needed rest, even though the race isn't even close to being finished. The wall is an interesting place. Some athletes hate it but I think I really like it. It's a turning point. For some athletes, it is even a breaking point, a point where they mentally decide to quit or give in to what they believe is an insurmountable task. It's almost like time stands still because you are so focussed on living in the moment. You have crossed a line with your body that few people ever get a chance to experience. It can be an addictive rush of adrenaline and if you love that sort of thing, I think that's what draws most triathletes back to experience. It's an interesting question to ask, "what am I made of today?" I am getting goose bumps just thinking about it again.

In 2012 at the full-distance World Championships in Hawaii, Mirinda Carfrae was poised to win her second World Championship title in typical fashion. She normally starts the run leg a few minutes behind the leaders and one by one, picks them off and passes them. As she approached Leanda Cave, her final competitor to overtake for the lead, Leanda turned to look at Mirinda as if to say, "Not this time, not today" and Leanda held off the attack with a charge of her own.

You could see at that very moment that she had broken Mirinda's confidence, her mental toughness and her belief that she could pass and overtake her. Mirinda would eventually fall back to finish in third place for the race. There are many video examples on YouTube that show athletes hitting their breaking points.

Pain is temporary. Quitting is forever. One of my favorite triathlon quotes is "You can quit and they won't care, but you will always know." I think of that quote a lot while I'm training because there are certainly days when you obviously can do your workouts, you just don't feel like it. Too many other things or as I like to say "other people's agendas for my life" are getting in the way. Daily choices are the stepping stones to developing mental toughness. You do whatever it takes to make it to the finish line each and every day.

When I coach kids in rowing, I like to tell them that when they are sitting in the starting gate of a race, the only thing that separates one boat from another is mental toughness. If you are all in similar boats, with similar ability and a similar race plan, the only thing left that can make a difference is mental toughness. You gain mental toughness by paying a price and depositing that experience into your mental memory bank. On race day, when it really matters, you get to make a withdrawal.

How do you win the mental struggle every day? The secret is in something I referred to earlier as your *Why Factor*. If your goal is to get up at 5:30 a.m. to attend a 6:00 a.m. spin class, you need to remember *why* you set that alarm in the first place. If you're a parent, it's likely because other people are counting on you to be heart healthy as you grow older. If you have children, being healthy and available to them when they re-ally need you should be your single best mo-tivator to get your butt out of bed and to get moving. Nobody plans on being a burden to others and yet that is normally the outcome of poor heart health daily choices. Old and sick is no way to live in your retirement.

Believe in yourself because anything is pos-sible for your life. Protect your dreams and don't let anyone discourage you from achieving them. People love to keep you grounded because of what they themselves may fear. I'm here to tell from my own per-sonal experience that anything is possible. You just have to believe and know *why* it is so important to you.

The Right Motivation

Why do people quit gym memberships? We've all been there. You join a
gym to lose weight and the next thing you
know you're not going any more. This is the
riddle that has perplexed the fitness industry
for years. I believe the problem is with immediate gratification. We have become a society that demands instant results. We all
want fast internet, fast service, fast food and
fast results in the gym. When we don't get
fast results, we move on to something else.

The right motivation inspires us to experience greatness, and motivation is what we
use to reason with ourselves to get out of
bed early every day and invest in our own
well-being. Motivation is the hard part until
you find your reason "*why*". Understanding
your W*hy Factor* is the magic bullet that
will propel you to a lifetime of good health.

From my earliest days in business, I learned
about the 80/20 rule. For heart healthy
adults, this rule would imply that 80 percent
of the population is in poor heart health and
that 20 percent have optimal heart health.
The actual numbers are more shocking. Ac-

cording to a recent study from the Heart Association of America a full 97 percent of adults in North America have sub-optimal heart health. Even worse, when polled, over 40 percent truly believed they did. Some of us just know we are not heart healthy but it's the ones who don't even realize it that really motivate me to educate as many people as possible about living heart healthy.

When I do presentations at local high schools, I always do an impromptu survey and the results are almost always the same. I ask students to put their hands up if either of their parents exercise once a week. I don't even qualify what type of exercise it might be. Usually I get half the kids putting their hands up. Then I ask whose parents exercise three times a week and most of the hands go down. I might have three or four remaining up now. Then I ask whose parents exercise six days a week and if anyone still has their hand up I ask what their parents do for exercise and the answer is always the same, they are a runners.

You don't have to be a distance runner or a triathlete to be heart healthy. You simply have to pick an activity you enjoy and find the right reasons for yourself to commit to doing it every day. I like non-impact activities like swimming, and spinning for adults because you can work in a group and reach your own individual pace using a heart rate monitor. No one gets dropped from a fast ride or a tough hill climb on a spin bike. All of these little factors go a long way in making the exercise experience enjoyable and that is part of the metal toughness you will need to continue exercising in the long run.

Joining a gym or exercise program with the sole purpose to lose the next ten pounds is a quick recipe for failure. Let's say you go to the gym and you work really hard for two months and you don't see the results on the scale. You think to yourself "why am I paying to do this?" You are working really hard with no visible results and so you stop going. The other outcome might be that you lose your target ten pounds but then what? What's your motivation now? Maybe you only had ten pounds to lose in the first place. Remember, skinny does not equal heart healthy.

There have been and will continue to be many new and wonderful fitness crazes. Hopefully you don't fall victim to all of the marketing hype, and that your will understand the purpose behind training you are doing.

In the beginning, I exercised out of a place of fear from the consequences of living an inactive lifestyle. Over time, I learned to enjoy exercising more because I discovered new activities that really served to inspire me. It was that daily feeling of accomplishment and reaching new goals that really started to change my belief system. My attitude became "why not me" instead of "why me?" The most important lesson that I can teach you is figuring out that your *Why Factor* has to be more powerful than any excuse you can come up with to quit or stay in bed. It's your million dollar question and your million dollar solution.

My "why" has taken me to Iron Distance triathlon finish lines twice and now my continuing journey has inspired me to serve people just like you. It's no fun being fit and healthy all alone, so I am finding new ways to coach more people to help them enjoy living heart healthy lives too.

Once I started focusing on daily heart health and not the scale, my weight just naturally adjusted to what it should be. My focus isn't on the weight any more, it's on *not* having to take cholesterol pills and heart medication. I really have no other choice if I want to stay off of medication. I have to decide to take care of my heart every day, and I don't want to even think of the consequences if I neglect to do so.

If I have to train in a heart healthy manner every day, I might as well learn to enjoy the experience. Racing in triathlons and being part of the triathlon community really lets me enjoy my training experience.

My son Warren did a sprint triathlon with me last summer and doing that together was priceless. How many dads get to have that kind of experience with their kids? I'm willing to bet not very many. This particular triathlon was held in one of our favorite places on Lake Muskoka. Our good friends offered to let us stay with them at their cottage for the weekend. Our sons had become friends years ago while attending a camp on the lake and we have remained good friends ever since. The experience that I got to share with Warren on that day was even better than finishing the full-distance triathlon finish line because it was an experience we got to share together and that is something that money can't buy.

When I talk about the right motivation, I ask people to challenge themselves to find their *Why Factor*. Your *Why Factor* is what you will use to reason with yourself to get out of bed every day to do your workout. In order for it to be effective, it needs to be very personal and so deeply motivating that you need it to happen as much as your body needs to draw its next breath. My race experiences continually change and that's what makes my sport fun and interesting, but my *Why Factor* never changes. I simply refuse to go on cholesterol and heart medication. It is a decision that I have to make every day. I need to feed my heart healthy activity every twenty-four hours to stay heart healthy. My body doesn't recognize weekends or holidays. I will typically run every day while on vacation. The point is that if you want to grow older and still feel like a million bucks, you have to keep deciding to invest in yourself every day.

Inspiration is the easy part. I'm inspired by the idea that I can continue to experience youthful activities with my family and friends. Just thinking about it gives me goose bumps. Motivation to get moving is the problem we all struggle with every day. I would be lying to you if I said I never want to take a day off, and to be honest, gaining new perspective and balance has allowed me to take the odd day off here or there if my body simply needs rest. I can usually tell it's time for an unscheduled rest day when I start getting cranky.

Typically, we struggle with our mind right before our workout even begins. This is the critical point where you start to reason with yourself that you should just stay in bed. You set your alarm clock for 5 a.m. or 6 a.m. with only the best of intentions and the next thing you know, there are 1000 voices in your head all screaming unanimously to hit the snooze button and go back to sleep. As exciting and inspiring as the thought of racing in a long distance triathlon can be, that event in and of itself is not enough to motivate me to get out of bed on a cold dark morning. For me, I have to remind myself every day that the first and only reason "WHY" I exercise is to stay heart healthy. Even though I am much healthier now than when I turned forty, I still consider myself high risk for relapse if I ever stop investing in my health every day.

On average, to do the activities I love, I went from not exercising at all to about forty-five minutes every day, to now any-

where from one hour to five hours of training a day depending where I am in my training plan. So why do it? Why do all the extra
training? If I stopped being a triathlete tomorrow, I would still need to train my heart
every day. The only thing that would change
is the duration and purpose of each workout.
What is it that people mentally need to have
to silence all of the excuses and just get out
of bed and do it?

The answer that I found can be summed up
in one word. I am motivated by the *experience* that I get to have because of the daily
work that I do. Experiences are the exciting
moments in life that I get to tell my friends
and family about. Nobody will want to hear
about all of the drudgery of training, they
want to hear about the excitement of swimming in the ocean with sharks and jellyfish
and coming face to face with a barracuda or
standing on the beach at the start of the race
right beside a two-time World Champion
and not having a clue who she was. You
don't know what you are going to discover,
who you are going to meet or what you are
going to find out about yourself until you
make a commitment and then go out and do
it. If you get excited just thinking about it,
the destination will be worth the journey.

I really believe that having unrealistic expectations is the primary reason why people quit exercising. People get frustrated and disappointed with the lack of results because they don't understand what results they should be focused on in the first place. People don't take the time to educate themselves about how their bodies work and then they don't select the right activities that will help them reach their goals.

We really do care about how others see us. We care about what they say and think of us. It is a basic human need that we strive to look good to others. A little knowledge with the right perspective helping you to make better choices can go a long way in achieving your desired outcome.

So if you can accept the fact that heart fit living is a process, and you follow the clues that other successful people leave for you to follow, then this book just might be the best thing to ever come into your life. Take a look around your world and find the groups of people that you would like to emulate and simply do what they do. If you want to have a killer beach volleyball body and the stamina to play all day, then this book and my free online tools can show you the way. If you want to go out and tackle a triathlon, you have also come to the right place, but please be aware that you will require more training knowledge than I have provided in these pages. The good news for you is that there are plenty of great coaching books and YouTube channels that can help you make sense of sport specific training along the way. The basic bones of every training system are pretty much the same and that is what I have shared with you today. More sport specific coaching comes at a price and it is usually worth every penny. Just make sure that everyone you are working with has the same purpose in mind. My daily coaching service which you can sign up for on my website is specifically designed to lock you into a 365 day commitment with yourself and I will remind you of your reasons for wanting a better life every day. A great coach provides you with perspective and options.

The best motivational aid for me is repetition. I watch the same coaching and training videos over and over again, just like watching a good movie, I look for clues or messages I might have missed the first fifty times I watched the video. Repetition reminds you to do two things: review your *Why Factor* every day, and to remember that other people are counting on you to be the healthiest you can be. It's all about making the right choices every day, and we could all use a little positive coaching in that department.

While my "Why Factor" hasn't changed over the past decade, my inspiration has. When I started this journey, my daughter was only 8 years old. She looked up to me and continued to do so until she hit those teen years. She trusted me, she liked me and she didn't mind my company at all.

When Katelyn started high school, she used to wait for the school bus and pray that I wouldn't ran past her bus stop in my running tights. That was simply mortifying to her. She spent the better part of her high school years locked away in her bedroom. She didn't want me to coach her high school rowing crew and that really hurt. She wanted to find her own way and create her own experiences and I had to respect that.

Katelyn is now in her final semester of high school and while I was out for my morning run the other day, Katelyn and her friends passed me in a car on their way to school. She rolled down her window and screamed "yah dad" despite my running tights. I guess I'm not an embarrassment after all.

Why Start Now?

Deciding to live heart healthy is a conscious daily choice. It is a life- long journey, not a destination alone. It is a journey of inspiring, being inspired, and understanding your own reasons *why* any of this really matters. Why should you care, and why should you start now? Choosing to invest in your heart health today is one of approximately 612 decisions you're probably going to make today, and really only one of the few that really matters. Living and feeling alive is about making good choices every day. Choose to spend one hour every day aimlessly surfing the net and you never get that time back. Choosing to spend that same hour actually *surfing,* and you never know where that decision to be active might take you. You will find that taking steps forward to making real and lasting change in your life is more of a mental process than a physical one. Most importantly, it is not too late to start. Now.

When I talk about fitness and daily heart health with people, I like to talk about the similarities between financial health and personal heart health because the same basic strategies apply to both. As an example of compounding benefits, I often ask people if they would like to retire at sixty with one million dollars in the bank. I go on to explain that if you saved one dollar a day from the day you were born until the day you turned sixty and averaged 8 percent interest, you would retire at sixty with five hundred-thousand dollars in the bank. If you paid a little more attention to your investment vehicle and averaged 9.7 percent return, you would retire at sixty with *one million dollars* in the bank. The beauty of compounding interest is that all the real benefits take place once your financial nest egg reaches critical mass (one million dollars). It is between the ages of forty and sixty when all the real magic and compounding benefits start to happen. If you continue to invest every day, it will continue to give you fantastic returns.

Let's say you're like me and you consider your house or your business as your financial retirement nest egg. Let's presume you don't have any retirement savings and you just turned forty. This is the time in many people's lives that if they do experience a financial windfall, likely due to an inheritance and not lottery tickets, they have a decision to make. Let's say you inherited one hundred fifty-six thousand dollars. You can invest the entire amount and start adding an additional dollar every day until you turn sixty using investment vehicles that yield an average rate of return of 9.7 percent and you will retire with one million dollars in the bank. Your other choice is to live for the moment, spend the money and find yourself right back where you started.

Your heart health works in about the same way. If you have led a sedentary lifestyle up until the time you turned forty, you can take comfort that you are no worse or different than most everyone else, but instead of feeling bad about the years that you could have been in better shape, start now and enjoy the years to come. The great thing is that like the potential of an inheritance, it's not too late to make significant changes in your forties. This is the time in your life when you are presented with options and your maturity and mastery of life or lack thereof will define who you are going to be. You can either accept the wisdom of successful people who have gone before you or you can continue down the same path you were already on. If you do what you've always done, you can expect the same results. Start making the right decision today.

I was once very much like you. I didn't need anyone to tell me that I needed to exercise or count calories, I knew that is important. I also knew it didn't matter what I'd done in the past, the only thing that mattered is what I chose to do that day. If you want to feel good about yourself today, all you need to do is get up and go for a walk. Move your body every day and good things are going to happen.

Inspiration is all around us. There are no shortages of inspiring stories about people who have faced incredible challenges in their lives only to push through what some would call barriers and succeed. Inspiration is the easy part; daily motivation is the hard part. You need to see the value that invest-ing forty-five to sixty minutes every day in your heart health is every bit as important as breathing, eating, drinking and sleeping. These are all things we do every day without even giving it a second thought. Deciding to invest in your heart health every day needs to be regarded in the same way and with the same sense of urgency.

For many of us and certainly for me, I had what I like to refer to as an "*uh-oh*" moment. This is when you can't ignore the warning signs any longer and you go to your doctor or the hospital to find out what has gone

wrong. The prescription after any life altering heart related event is normally diet, exercise, and/or medication. When I realized the
alternative was to be on medication the rest
of my life, I started making small decisions
that eventually culminated in a completely
different lifestyle with health benefits I
could only dream of before.

I started this journey of investing in myself
by walking and jogging for forty-five
minutes (5k) every day, seven days a week
because I needed to make my heart healthier. Over time, I simply decided that I
wanted to experience more from my life. If
you decide that you want to experience
more, you're going to need to do more. It's
that easy (or that hard), depending on your
point of view.

The challenge most people face, believe it or
not, is fear. People fear loss. "What if I can't
eat the foods I love any more, or what if I
have to get up an hour early and lose that
hour of sleep?" People also fear the process.
"I hate running, I know my body will be
sore, I don't feel fit enough to join a gym."
Aside from fear, some people are paralyzed
by a less than desirable outcome. "What if I
work really hard for thirty or sixty days and
I don't see the results I wanted on the

scale?" Part of being successful in life is learning how to manage fear.

Living heart healthy is part of a daily decision making process. If this is the only page you read in this book, your strategy for heart healthy living is to go for a moderately paced walk every day for forty-five minutes, and start today. Personally, however, I reasoned that if I was going to do something every day, I really needed better motivation to enjoy it, and as my belief system changed, my expectations for myself changed as well. The critical difference is that I followed my decision up with action and didn't delay any longer.

Life is a process, and at every stage, we enter with a certain level of maturity. To be successful, we enter the next stage with both maturity and mastery over the previous challenges. Working with parents in their forties is very special to me because not only are you my peers, you're at the stage in life when you're mature enough to know better, and still young enough to care.

Welcome to the community of heart healthy living, it's one of those things in life that money can't buy. Admittance has to be earned.

Why Not Me?

Instead of asking, "why me?" ask yourself, "why not me?" Somebody has to be the role model in your circle of family and friends, the person your kids look up to when life knocks you down. Ask yourself not what you will be but who you will be and start being that person today. If you want your family and friends to look up to you for inspiration, then live an inspired life. Don't wait for someone to give you permission. Start living the life you want to live today.

My high school English teacher Mrs. Kerman will be thrilled and surprised to see that not only can I write a book and tell an interesting story but that I have been asked to be a contributing writer for online health and wellness publications. Instead of saying, "I can't write because I am not a writer," I asked the question, "how do I tell a compelling story and what are my next steps?" This book may never become a bestseller or win a literary prize but by putting my story out there to the world, it helps to serve others and that's what really matters.

In college, we were taught in our marketing program that success can be found in products or services that serve the masses. Identify a common problem that many people share and then provide a solution that you believe in 100 percent. According to a recent study conducted by the American Heart and Lung Association, most adults in North America (97 percent) do not have optimal heart health and will have a higher than average probability of being negatively affected by heart disease. That is a *huge problem*! The opportunity can be found by asking the question, "How can I serve these people so they can make better decisions for their lives? How can I motivate them to experience life living heart healthy?"

Fortunately for you, the answers are simple enough and can be found right here in this book.

Sometimes in life we can feel trapped or caged by the reality we create for ourselves in our own mind. We put up barriers to our own success and we learn to live our life comfortably adverse to fear and risk. These people are merely existing. These people are simply punching the clock of time until their time is up.

There is an open door to leave the cage at any time and what is on the other side of that door is work. If you want to be the person your kids need you to be, embrace that work every day. You won't be paid financially for all of the hard work you do but you will be rewarded with a richness that only healthy living can buy. Why not you, indeed. Get up an hour early every day and choose who you are going to be.

Eating Well Makes You Feel Good

Food! I love to eat. I have cravings just like everyone else. I don't buy chips because I have no willpower. As much as I grew up on soda and chips, you would think by now that I would know better and I do, but I still get those cravings and the key is not to have those foods in the house in the first place so you won't have to have as many battles with yourself.

The food I have come to love is what I call "real food." That is, food that is as natural as possible with the least amount of processing. Wherever I go, no matter what city I am in there is always a farmers market. As much as the grocery store is convenient and cheap, there is something special about running past a farmer's field, asking what fresh produce they have available and returning later in the day for a fresh picked basket just for you. What you do next with them is up to you but I like to keep an open mind to new foods and new flavors.

Spartan diets SUCK! Anything that starts with the words "You can't eat…" is no way to go through life. Common sense, moderation and learning to make better choices are better guides. So many people get caught up in fancy diet programs, and some people even count points instead of food. Diet marketing companies do have success with their programs and I remember sitting down with a good friend a few years back who was raving about the success of her new weight loss program. She was even allowed to eat three whole chicken wings as a treat because they were worth a certain number of "points" that her diet told her she was allowed to have. I don't know about you but I count points in football games and basketball games, not when I'm eating food. What I'm trying to say here is you need to understand more about the foods you are eating. You need to understand calories per serving, sodium, fibre and sugar content. In other words, you need to learn to read a food label.

Knowledge helps you make better choices. Have you ever been to a birthday party and where the women are offered a piece of cake they say "no thank you," or, "just a little piece for me thanks?" I love going to those parties because when someone asks me if I want a piece of cake, I say "absolutely! And while you're at it, give me what they don't want and I will eat that too." I know that piece of cake certainly must contain 800 to 1000 calories. I also know that I will burn about 800 fat burning calories in a sixty minute endurance spin class. When you understand how calories work, it's not a big deal at all to have your cake and eat it too. The trick is knowledge and balance. You can't eat like that every day, but once a month won't kill you either. If you completely deprive yourself from the foods you love eating, then you will never feel happy about your life. You will always fear the loss of the foods you love and that mind game will wreak havoc with your daily mental battles. It's not about punishing yourself or beating yourself up every day. It's about putting your life into perspective and making the best choices so that you can live with yourself with the outcome. Am I going to enjoy a piece? You bet! Am I always going to have a second piece? Not likely. Am I going to eat cake every day or every week? No. Am I going to beat myself up when I do eat a piece? No way! I invest in myself every day so that I can enjoy living.

I am a marketer by trade and what diet marketing companies do is called "packaging". Someone has taken basic information about food and packaged it in a way that looks like the easy, sure- fire road to success.

I prefer a more common sense approach to my food choices and that comes from experience and having perspective. I want my cake and I want to eat it too. I love birthday cake or any cake for that matter. There is a local bakery here in my home town that is famous for their moist delicious cakes and buttery cream fudge frosting. I love it!   Wash it down with a cold glass of milk and embrace the sugar coma that follows.

When you live with balance, you are more likely to stick with clean eating because you won't feel deprived all of the time. What I have noticed is that I don't gorge myself anymore. Now, when I eat comfort foods, I do so with the knowledge of how my body works and how my body will consume, process, and burn off those calories.

What exactly is clean eating? Essentially, clean eating is about eating foods that have not been highly processed, or eating foods that are as close to their natural form as possible. You try to limit your ingredient list to ingredients that occur more naturally, even organically where possible. For example, you can't ban sugar from your diet because it is a naturally found ingredient in fruits but refined sugar which is highly processed should be limited or avoided altogether.

When you start eating six smaller "clean" meals a day, your stomach starts to shrink and you feel fuller faster. The good news is that this feeling of fullness helps you to walk away from the table sooner.

One of the many things my parents taught me as a young boy was to have manners, especially at the dinner table. Things like never eat at the table with your hat on; always wash your hands before you eat and always help with the dishes after a meal. My grandmother would cook for hours making the best homemade pierogie's, and after the meal, because she had no dishwasher, we would all help out cleaning the table and washing the dishes. As a parent, I have tried to raise my kids with the same manners. I have shown them how to set a proper table for supper and they know enough that when I start to clear the table, that is their cue to join in.

These basic values help guide my controlled eating habits. The next time you eat at a large family gathering, be the one to get up first and start clearing dishes. Take note of who remains at the table with their plate to polish off any remaining food on the table. The next visual clue of an overeater is watching people disappear to the couch into a food coma inspired nap.

Being the first to start clearing the table signals to your brain that it's time to stop eating. Even if I don't get up immediately, I start stacking other people plates onto mine ensuring I won't be tempted to put a little more onto my plate.

When I eat at someone else's home, I don't ask questions such as, "is there any butter in this" or "what kind of oil did you use because I only eat extra virgin olive oil?" I eat a little bit of everything and go back for seconds on the lean protein or vegetables.

When my mother or mother-in-law tells me to sit down and don't worry about the dishes, I know better. I am doing it as much for myself as I am doing it out of respect for them. When people entertain, they tend to make too much food and then encourage you to polish it off because they don't want any leftovers. That's their problem, not yours.

Feeling good about eating food reaches far beyond the physical act of consuming it. You can feel good about where you buy your fresh local ingredients. You can feel good about teaching your kids life skills such as how to cook. You can feel good about eating comfort foods that are laden with fatty ingredients and you can feel good about yourself when you pitch in to help clean up the meal.

People who fail to utilize proper nutritional habits fear losing the foods they have grown to love. They fear that loss so much that they don't even try other approaches to eating. Taking control is key, and it does not mean a lifetime of depriving yourself of foods you love. As you change your habits, your desires change for the better foods. When I control my actions, I am less likely to give into temptations.

At home, I have my pantry of ingredients that get mixed and combined to create a variety of healthy food flavors and options. I try to eat six healthy meals every day and that typically consists of steel cut oats for breakfast, yogurt and fruit for a snack, spinach salad with quinoa for lunch, almond butter and jam sandwich for a snack, a lean protein and vegetable meal for dinner and then a bowl of commercially made cereal for a pre-bedtime snack. Generally, that is what my food intake looks like every day combined with about six full glasses of water and some skim milk. I always drink a glass of chocolate milk as a post workout recovery drink (science backs it and it works for me). There is a tone of controversy online about chocolate milk so you can choose the best post workout drink to suit your needs.

When it comes to eating food, I tend to look at my plate and assess whether I have a lean protein, a vegetable or a carbohydrate and how much of each I have on my plate. The only one of the three categories that concerns me is the carbohydrates because they will quickly turn to sugar in my bloodstream and if I don't engage in regular daily training, that sugar will turn into unwanted fat. I can visualize what six ounces of protein looks like so that is easy to gauge (about the size of two decks of cards).

When you eat reasonably "clean" like this consistently for six days in a row, it's OK to take a night off and eat whatever you like so long as it's not the norm.

I live in wine country and I am close enough to the vineyards that from August through November I can hear the bangers that keep the birds at bay from stealing the farmers fall harvest. It is a constant reminder that I live in an area that is based on agriculture and farming fresh foods. There are so many talented chefs who can create the most amazing meals, and yet the best meals normally come from simple quality fresh ingredients. One of my favorite chefs often says that a recipe is only a starting point, merely a suggestion and the rest comes from your own inspiration. I am inspired by fresh food and fresh, crisp, clean flavors.

Consider cooking as part of a richer life experience that makes up the person who you want to be. Being knowledgeable makes you more interesting as a person. It gives you something to talk about other than yourself. People often want to know what it feels like to finish a full-distance triathlon, and while I am happy to tell them stories, I would rather find more common ground such as cooking and eating (a need we all share) and explore common interests together. Being too self-absorbed in your life's accomplishments can become boring rather quickly to anyone who does not share the same experience.

I had a great conversation the other day with my auto mechanic whom I hadn't seen in a few years. I was sitting in his office waiting for a repair to be completed, and being only five weeks away from my next race, I wanted to rub my clean eating and exercising lifestyle in his chain- smoking face. I like Mark and I know he could care a less about my "healthy bad habits" as he calls them. What I did notice on his desk was that he was reading an article about the pros and cons of a "Gluten Free" diet. So rather than talking in a one sided conversation about heart healthy living, I engaged him in a conversation about eating "Gluten Free." Turns out he has been on a gluten free diet now for several years and it was interesting to hear what he had to say. There I was, the triathlete learning about healthy eating from the chain smoker. Common ground encourages conversation and opinion.

I had another great conversation with a client at my spin studio who is a vegan. I started asking her all kinds of questions and the funny thing was that she got all defensive. She said most people normally attack her point of view but she sensed I really was interested. I will never be a vegan but I am much closer to a vegetarian than a pure meat eater. When you take the time to listen to others and respect their point of view, you become more interesting as a person and more people will open up to you. Again, life is about having perspective and recognizing and respecting that we are all free to make

our own choices so long as we can live with
the outcomes.

When you open your mind, eyes, and ears to
others, it's amazing what common ground
you might find. Talking about food makes
me feel good. Learning about food makes
me feel good and of course eating food
makes me feel good. When my chatty
daughter was five years old, I told her to
close her pie hole, and she ran crying to her
mother. She said, "Daddy says I can't talk
anymore." So the next time someone tells
you to "close your pie hole" it may not mean
they want you to stop eating, they might just
want you to talk less and to listen more to
what they have to say. Be a good listener.

Fat Loss vs Water Loss

The human body metabolizes fat and ex-
cretes it as 17% waste by-product and 83%
carbon dioxide. In order to lose one pound
of fat in one week, you need to consume
3500 fewer calories than you burn. In order
to metabolize fat, you need to get your heart
rate into the aerobic zone. Once you have all
of the facts about your diet and exercise, you
will start to understand the science and facts
behind weight management.

I choose to believe that deep down inside we
are all intelligent and reasonable people.
When people come into my indoor cycling
studio and announce after one month that
they have lost twenty or more pounds, it's
hard not to be happy and excited for them
but the reality is that they have set themselves up for failure. Our bodies are made
up of between 55 percent and 60 percent water. If you have ever actually seen what a
twenty pound bag of fat looks like, you will
realize quickly that it is highly unlikely that
you were able to metabolize and shed all of
that fat in thirty one days.

More likely than not, if you have been exercising six days a week and consuming fewer calories than you expend every day, you have probably shed two to five pounds of fat and the rest of the weight loss can be attributed to water loss.

When I did my first full-distance triathlon race in Louisville, my body shed over eight litres of water that day. Eight litres of water represents about twenty pounds. During the race, I consumed approximately four to five litres of water and electrolyte sports drinks, replacing ten pounds of the water lost, leaving me with a net loss of ten pounds on race day. Any reasonable person will be able to argue very successfully that the human body cannot shed ten pounds of fat in one day, so quick weight loss must be water loss resulting from dehydration.

I went to my butcher the other day and asked him to collect ten pounds of animal fat for me. I wanted to show the folks at my cycling studio what ten pounds of fat actually looks like and ask how anyone could reasonably expect to metabolize that kind of thing off of their bodies in such a short period of time. Water loss I can believe, but actual fat? I'm not buying it. If you exercise good eating habits with regular exercise over a long enough period of time, you will lose weight.

When it comes to exercising, we need to keep things simple if we want to experience long term success. A great saying I hear around triathlon circles is that we didn't create the bodies we have in one day; we haven't lived our lives in one day, so why should anyone believe that they can get fit or lose a tremendous amount of weight in one day or even thirty days. People often tell me they will give it a try for three months to which I reply what is your measurement of success after three months. If people expect to lose anything more than two pounds a month, I would like to see the math in their diet and fitness plan that will support their end goal.

Weight management is simple math. Consume fewer calories than you expend and you will lose weight. Not many people are disciplined enough to follow through with that paperwork so they end up ultimately disappointed or frustrated when they see large weight gains or losses. For that reason, I am asking you to throw your scale away. If you are open to the idea of learning how to work out aerobically and understand how your body consumes food for fuel, and you are disciplined enough to follow your plan, you will be able to manage your weight to whatever weight makes you feel confident and good about yourself.

There is no such thing as an "ideal" weight. We come in all shapes and sizes. For me, ultimate fitness comes down to being heart healthy enough to participate in any youthful activity I choose. I consider myself to be an average triathlete. I'm not the fastest or the slowest. I am happily seeded right in the middle. My expectations are that I can finish any race that I enter. If the stars are aligned and I have an exceptional and well prepared training season, I might be able to pull off a higher place finish. Your only real goal is to be prepared enough to experience that finish line successfully and with a smile on your face. The race is just the cherry on top of the cake. In this case you get to enjoy the entire cake too.

You can watch my four minute video and decide for yourself if you think you could shed that kind of mass in thirty days or less. Just visit the Dave Buzanko YouTube channel and look for the fat loss vs water loss in the Hearfit365 Q & A section.

Daily Calories

Being a long distance triathlete, I need to understand how my body consumes fat and sugar for fuel. This is so important for you to understand too because if your desire is to maintain a healthy weight, you are going to need a basic understanding of the cause and effect relationship between food and daily training to achieve your goals. When people train or exercise in the aerobic zone (60 percent - 80 percent of my maximum heart rate) during activities such as endurance swimming, cycling and jogging, your body is consuming fat for fuel and this is where we see long term weight management occur.

At certain times, some of the activities you do will take you into the anaerobic zone (80 percent - 95 percent of my maximum heart rate).This occurs during activities which require short bursts at maximum effort, such as playing team sports like hockey and basketball or strength fitness classes.

When you are in the anaerobic heart rate zone, your body can't process the fat quickly enough so it burns the sugar in your bloodstream for fuel. This is why so many runners or endurance athletes carb load before a big race. They want to have the right mix of fat and sugar in their body to help fuel them for their race. Marathon runners tend to settle into a heart rate of 80 to 85 percent depending on how hard they are pushing themselves on race day and they need sugar in their bloodstream to fuel their race. Once your body settles into the anaerobic heart rate zone (after about sixty minutes for most distance runners), you stop burning fat for fuel because at that heart rate, it's easier for your body to break down lean muscle mass for fuel than fat. This is why runners will drink flat cola and eat orange slices and performance gels during a race. These food sources all represent liquid sugar and an immediate source of fuel for their body to consume. What goes in gets immediately burned off.

As a typical adult who is looking to maintain a healthy heart and healthy weight, your objective is to look at food as fuel. Weight management is a simple mathematical exercise of calories in vs. calories out. But remember that all calories and all sweat are not created equal. The 500 calories in a spinach salad are completely different from the 500 calories in a hamburger. You would need to eat seventy-five cups of spinach to equal the calories in one quarter pound hamburger with cheese. The nutrients in spinach are the building blocks of life. The nutrients in a cheeseburger are hardeners for your arteries.

One cheeseburger won't kill you but eating one every day just might. Just as the 800 calories burned in an endurance spin class are different from the 800 calories burned in a strength spin class. If the purpose of your workout is to burn fat, then the right training for you is fifteen minutes of core resistance training followed by endurance. If your purpose is to build muscle, then strength training is right for you. We all have something called Glycogen in our blood stream and that is the available sugar your body burns for fuel when you work out. You have about fifteen to thirty minutes worth to burn through before your body starts consuming fat for fuel. Understanding the differences between the types of exercises you do, the heart rates you will be training at along with the types of calories you consume and burn is the basic knowledge you need for living life as a heart healthy adult.

Why do people quit or stop taking action to improve their lives? Mostly it's because people fear losing something they have grown to love. They fear the process of the work and pain involved in making real change and they fear that the outcome may not be what they had originally desired. People fear loss, fear the process, or fear the potential of pain, so they quit.

It is easy to blame others for what you don't know or don't understand. Your job, if you want to be a better you is to start understanding and learning the simple process for long term significant change. Most people quit a fitness program because they don't achieve the result they are looking for and that is typically weight loss. When people don't feel the immediate gratification from the scale tipping in the right direction, they give up in frustration when in reality, a basic understanding of how your body works is all they really need to achieve success with any physical activity on a daily basis.

I have worked with many adult women between the ages of twenty-five and sixty, and what I often see in overweight women is that they desperately want to lose an unrealistic amount of weight in an unrealistic amount of time.

People tend to make quick decisions based on what the scale is telling them on any given day. While it's true that bigger people have more weight to lose, they too will hit a wall where they stop seeing the large amount of monthly weight loss and when that happens, they typically get discouraged and quit. Most of the weight loss you see on the scale on a daily basis is simply fluctuation in hydration. Weight loss occurs when you burn more calories on a monthly basis than you consume.

Ask any rower or wrestler or any athlete that needs to make weight for a competition and they will tell you the easiest way to drop ten pounds in one day is to do a sweat run. I lose twenty pounds of water in a single day when I compete in a full-distance triathlon. I don't shed fat, I lose water, water that needs to get back into my system with appropriate hydration following my race.

I am here to tell you that non-impact endurance work performed six days a week for forty-five minutes a day is all you need to build a strong heart, reduce your risk of cardiovascular diseases, and maintain a healthy weight. Losing two pounds a month consistently is terrific success and building a strong heart is even better. It took me five years to lose fifty pounds and I did it in a safe and intelligent way.

Once you understand your daily calorie consumption and burn, you start to see where success and failure can be found. Refer to my free Community Heartfit Wellness Program found on the heartfit365.com website for a free download to start mapping out a plan for weight management. This is really just an eye opening exercise to give you more detailed perspective into your eating and exercise habits. In order for you to make the best possible choices for your health, wouldn't you agree that you need to have all of the facts before you go out and spend your hard earned money on gym memberships or at the grocery store? An informed consumer is a smart consumer, and smart consumers usually get the best results.

What I wish I knew 30 years ago about sugar: Not all calories are created equal. Added sugar is more problematic than you might think. It is 8x more addictive than Cocaine and has been linked to cancer and tumor growth. For more information about added sugar in your diet, please watch the videos on the SUGAR page at Heartfit365.com.

Heartfit Training – A Simple Plan to Follow

So how can you get started? What are your first steps? For me, step one is as simple as understanding WHY I need to do something good for my heart every day. Step two is setting a goal.

A goal is defined by having a certain quantifiable outcome within a certain period of time. Saying "I would like to lose ten pounds" is a wish or a desire at best. Saying, "I will lose ten pounds in ten months" is a quantifiable goal with an associated time line. There is a beginning, an ending, and a result. I don't like to focus on weight goals too much. I found better success focussing on daily heart fit goals and once I began to understand how my body consumes food for fuel, if I wanted to lose weight, I simply consumed fewer calories than I expended. My current goal is to do some form of heart healthy activity for at least one hour every morning. I usually surpass that time every day but it is the only goal I need to keep moving forward.

For you, the best advice I can give you is to throw away your scale and purchase a wireless heart rate monitor. I have set up a link from my Heartfit365.com website to show you the exact model I have used for the past five years and it can be purchased if you wish directly through the Amazon website link.

Here is the goal that I recommend for anyone who would like to be heart healthy. Do any type of aerobic activity at your target heart rate (75 percent of max) for a minimum of forty-five minutes, six days a week. Take one day off for rest. It's that simple.

This is a simple and proven formula for success. With little more than an old pair of running shoes and a list of foods that were high in cholesterol to avoid, this daily goal turned my life around and it is easy enough that anyone reading this book can follow my same path. Ever since I started focussing on my daily heart health and stopped worrying about my weight, the weight started gradually disappearing and my cholesterol went down as a direct result of doing and eating the right things for my body. You can't out exercise a bad diet-for weight loss.
I have a history in my family of high cholesterol and heart disease so while I may be

predisposed to certain risk factors, my focus is on controlling what I can and that is having a healthy heart.

Figuring out your target heart rate for the average adult is simple math. If you become more serious about athletics and desire more accurate calculations, your best bet is to pay to have a Lactate Threshold test or a VO2 test done by a professional testing facility. For the rest of us, this simple formula will do just fine. For men, the calculation is 220 – your age x 75 percent. For women, the calculation is 226 – your age x 75 percent. The aerobic zone actually falls between 60 percent and 80 percent of your maximum heart rate so I like to advise people to strive for 75 percent. That number allows you to work hard enough to get the maximum aerobic benefits without crossing the anaerobic threshold. You can track your heart rate manually but that is like taking the speedometer out of your car. You can guess how fast you are going or how hard you are working but it is only a guess at best. I prefer to use Timex road trainer heart rate monitor.

There is a difference between aerobic and anaerobic exercise, and not understanding the difference is why many do not reach their fitness goals. Have you ever joined a gym or bought a piece of fitness equipment only to quit the gym or have that expensive gym equipment become an unused reminder that you can be an impulse buyer? I struggled with bad decisions too and I still have a stair climber collecting dust in my basement.

Knowledge, repetition and persistence are the keys to thriving in a fitness program that you can sustain and enjoy. I like the idea of non-impact activities for adults because by the time we hit thirty-five, we have pretty much abused our bodies. Choosing non-impact activities like swimming, cycling, and rowing are great ways to exercise your heart while incurring very little wear and tear to your body. What's more, with non-impact activities, your body requires less recovery time between workouts so it would be safe and easy to do a combination of these activities six days a week. You will notice that I left off walking, jogging, and running from my list. This is because these activities when done at the correct intensity are considered impact activities and will wear your body down quicker and require longer recovery periods.

As a triathlete, I combine a minimum of three swim, bike and run workouts every week while only training six days a week. A quick and simple calculation reveals that this is nine workouts in six days. I am often required to do multiple workouts in a day, but when you train with purpose, your training plan allows for adequate time and rest between certain training sessions.

For example, I would not run three days in a row, then bike three days in a row and throw in the odd swim session where time permits. Every training session has to have a purpose. Without a clear sense of purpose, you are simply exercising and increasing the likelihood that your end goal will not be reached or that will incur a goal stopping injury.

If I was totally new to fitness and I wanted to make the most significant impact on my heart health, I would join a facility that had a pool for lane swimming, an indoor running track or at the least multiple treadmills and indoor cycling equipment (not necessarily classes). I would purchase a heart rate monitor and do the simple target heart rate calculation from the previous pages. Next I would get active in any one of those three mentioned activities every morning at 6 a.m. and knock that forty-five minute workout out of the park! Be careful not to do running workouts back to back on consecutive days.

You want to space those workouts out to reduce the wear and tear and allow for adequate rest for your body.

If you wanted to join an indoor cycling facility that only offers classes, make sure that
they use heart rate monitors and heart rate
training as their guiding philosophy. The
SPINNING® program was built on this philosophy and as a triathlete; this is what drew
me to become certified as a SPINNING®
Instructor. The unfortunate part is that not
every instructor or facility recognizes the
importance of heart rate training so do your
homework before you put your money
down. Take a class and if the instructor stays
in the saddle and seems more concerned
about getting a good workout in for him or
herself, this is usually a good indication that
you are in the wrong place.

Indoor cycling in my opinion is the perfect
activity for most adults. It's great to see people being active outside, but with all of the
stops, cars, and other road hazards, indoor
cycling just makes a lot of sense. I own a
small spinning studio called Tri Cycling Stu-
dios® and we have thirty bikes. All of my in-
structors are triathletes and they all understand the importance of heart rate training. A
great instructor understands that they are at

the studio to coach you and help you. They are not supposed to be there for their own workout.

What I love the most about indoor cycling is that families and couples can spin together. Once you understand the basics, you are there for a forty-five minute endurance ride and because you comprehend the purpose of each workout, it is an inclusive activity that you can do with others of varying abilities. When you understand the progression of how one workout builds on the next, your training sessions begin to take on purpose, meaning and enjoyment.

Some people join the trend of the month camps that offer high intensity anaerobic workouts and have lots of variety, yet yield mixed results and leave a lot of people in their forties bruised, sore and even more dis-couraged. What I can tell you with confi-dence is that there is an Order of Operation to how your body works to burn calories when you are working out for sixty minutes. As mentioned previously, you want to do strength training first for fifteen to twenty minutes to burn up the Glycogen in your bloodstream (this is the available sugar that your body fuels itself on at the beginning of your workout). Once all of the glycogen has been depleted, your body will consume fat for fuel only if you are working in the aerobic zone. Drinking a sports drink during this hour introduces more available sugar as a fuel source and limits your body's ability to burn fat for fuel. Water is your best hydration option for sixty minute workouts.

There are two distinct differences between aerobic and anaerobic activities and what your body experiences with each. As a full-distance triathlete, I am keenly aware that if I don't pay close attention to my body, specifically my heart rate, not only am I unlikely to finish the race but I could also die due to organs shutting down during the race.

When you are working aerobically (this is known as the fat burning zone) your body consumes fat for fuel. It is an accepted fact that the fat burning zone sits between 60 percent and 80 percent of your maximum heart rate. When you are wearing a heart rate monitor, you get immediate feedback that tells you whether you are working too hard, too little or just right. Most people who exercise use "perceived exertion" as their guide and as we discussed earlier, that is not a very accurate or efficient measuring gauge. Wearing a heart rate monitor keeps you honest and informed about your efforts.

Examples of aerobic activities would be flat cross-country skiing, aerobic dancing, swimming, bicycling, jogging, elliptical training, or rowing.

When you are working anaerobically (this is known as the strength building zone) your body consumes sugar for fuel. Going anaerobic generally means your heart rate is at 80 percent of your maximum heart rate or higher. Anaerobic sports include but are not limited to basketball, hockey, stair climbing and mountain bike riding. During these activities you have short bursts of intense activity followed by a much needed recovery period. The great thing about going anaerobic is that it is a self- limiting activity. You can only go for short bursts before your heart and lungs rebel against you forcing you to stop.

For people who choose not to exercise, those sugar stores (high calorie meals and snacks) quickly turn to fat and before too long, you have gained more than a few extra unwanted pounds. The unfair part of this equation is that you can pack on calories a whole lot faster than you can burn them off.

As a teen growing up, I was constantly getting pounding headaches while playing
sports. My Doctor told me I had a condition
called low blood sugar. His advice was to
have a sugary drink on the side lines while I
played sports. You can imagine how thrilled
and understanding my high school football
teammates were when after or even during
wind sprints, if I was developing a headache, I had a pass to get a drink of soda from
our trainer on the sidelines. My days playing
football were numbered and I chose to play
sports with less intimidation and more drink
breaks like basketball and baseball. Eventually as I became a young adult, the headaches became fewer and I eventually forgot
all about them because as a young father, I
was becoming more and more inactive. I
wasn't playing sports any more, I was sup-
porting my kids who were playing sports.

As an adult at around the age of thirty-five, I
began to play pick-up hockey with all of the
men on my wife's side of the family. Even
today at forty-eight, I play our regular game
of pick-up hockey every Thursday night at
10 p.m. followed by a couple of beers at the
bar afterwards. Something that also started
occurring on a regular basis the morning after hockey was that I would have a slight
headache for about an hour after I woke up

on Friday mornings. I attributed this to a slight hangover from being dehydrated from playing hockey and then drinking beer to re-hydrate. This is what is referred to as "old time hockey."

At the start of this year's triathlon training season, two of my training partners and I decided that we would do a full-distance race together in Cozumel Mexico. We knew that race day was likely to be hot and humid and that flat cola would be a staple for fuel on the race course. A wise triathlete practices both the activity and the nutrition to be used during the race so that the body is conditioned for what you will put into it on race day.

I decided that I was going to train with cola on my runs instead of plain water and gels and that decision to use liquid sugar in the form of flat cola in my training has contributed to my fastest race times to date. I was thinking about hockey and those pesky headaches on Friday mornings and at the start of this season, I began drinking a can of soda on the way to the rink every Thursday night. While the soda does make you gassy, the headaches have been completely absent this season. I took a simple problem from my past and combined it with what I now know about how my body works today and utilized it for success in my sporting activities. I am most definitely not sitting around drinking soda all day. In fact, I focus on drinking six to eight glasses of plain water every day to stay hydrated. I now know that liquid sugar does play a role in my ability to perform better in sports where my body is searching for and burning sugar in the blood stream for fuel. Armed with this new perspective on heart rates and choices for hydration, my outcomes have been decidedly more successful.

A Personal Journey

Gaining a healthy new perspective has allowed me to share many stories about my personal journey and my transformation from being an overweight and out of shape dad to becoming a full-distance triathlete.

While not every reader will be inspired to follow in my footsteps and take on triathlon, my hope is that you will look at your life as a journey, much like I have with the best adventures still left to come.

They say that completing a full-distance triathlon is not so much about crossing the finish line as it is about the people you meet and the experiences you get to have along the way. When I look back at my life so far, I can see many twists and turns, many highs and lows and Truly, it's not the stuff that I have accumulated that's important, it's the people I've met and served and the experiences we've shared.

A good friend of mine is the VP of Human Resources for a very large company and in her politically correct way, she likes to point out that I'm not different, I'm "unique".

That's a very polite way of saying one day I might grow up.

I've had the traditional jobs and I've experienced life as an entrepreneur and I much prefer the latter. Many of you who are reading this book are working at traditional jobs with traditional responsibilities and there is nothing wrong with that at all. The only difference between you and me is how I prioritize my hours every day.

I have often used the phrase that I like to "lead by example." I would much rather show you how to do what needs to be done than talk about it. I know what you're thinking…if you've read this this far, I've been telling you what to do for a while now.

A great coach doesn't tell you what to do. A great coach is a good listener. They listen, offer you perspective and say if you choose this activity, then this might happen. If you choose this other activity, then this other thing might happen.

What is an example of better choices you could make for yourself today?

As an adult, you should be getting seven to eight hours of sleep each night. If you are going to get up at 5:30 a.m. to work out at 6 a.m., that means you will need to start going to bed between 10 p.m. and 11 p.m. That's lights out mister, no TV while trying to go to sleep. This is simply a choice you get to make every day. I have been doing this for a few years now and really, what am I missing? I have several news sources at my disposal throughout the day so no need to catch the 11 p.m. news. The kids are normally settled by 9:30 p.m. so that gives my wife and me an hour or so to decompress on the couch together before heading off to bed. You can't burn the candle at both ends and expect there not to be any negative consequences. Rest is a very important part of recovery and if you are going to start training with aerobic purpose, your body will thrive on that extra hour of rest.

You may not ever cross a triathlon finish line and that's ok. So what are some of the other ways that living heart healthy can affect your journey in life?

As an example of how heart healthy living has altered my life's experiences, something I had always wanted to do and never had the chance to do as a young boy was canoe in

Algonquin Park. The park is located in Central Ontario, and since I was a young boy, I always wanted to camp in the remote interior woods overnight. When my son was only five years old, I decided to take a leap of faith and take him on a father and son camping trip into the park. I had no idea what I was doing, but my wife's uncle was a Boy Scout Leader and he was happy to give me a few pointers about packing my canoe and food and surviving in the woods.

Since that first weekend, it has become an annual tradition as a father and "kids" camping trip. At one point we were up to eight dads and seventeen kids. The girls have taken over in numbers on the kid's side and for us dads with daughters, it has made for a very special annual trip. No boys, no moms: no blood, no foul, and we all have a great time every year. This is a weekend the kids always talk about and look forward to experiencing every year. It is actually a very cool trip. The kids do a lot of growing up over that weekend. They get to do things that their moms would never agree to, but they are always safe and they get to push their own boundaries of comfort and limitations. Just around the time I started training for my first triathlon, I was so rigid in my training and so focussed on not missing a single training day, I decided to bring my training gear up to the park with me. I knew that my kids would be safe in our tent if I headed out for a training session because there were lots of dads there to help out if needed.

The neat thing was that year after year more of the dads and kids started to join in on the swimming, the biking and the running in the park. Those activities completely changed my experience of camping in the park. What was started as a bit of a routine are now anticipated highlights of the weekend.

Before long we had four dads joining in on sunrise rides across the park where I have experienced possibly one of the most amazing sunrises I have ever seen. I still get a kick out of recalling a ride with my friend Mike who sports a few extra pounds around the midsection. When you are riding through Algonquin Park, it seems like one never ending hill climb on the bike and the downhill's are always way too short. The routine was that my "cycling" friends would attack the hills while I would simply spin through them. Inevitably we would all reach the top, usually together, but after the first hour of riding, fitness started to play a role and those cyclists who were not as fit were starting to play catch-up after the bigger hill climbs. I remember one downhill in particular when I thought we had left Mike in the dust on the climb and then all of a sudden he went screaming by us on the descent. I will never forget what he said as he passed us. He yelled out "fat guys win" and then he laughed with his distinctive chuckle. Mike is not in the same physical condition that I am in and yet he hung in there for the whole ride and he was having just as much fun as the rest of us. What I love about being phys-ically active; it brings out the best and usu-ally the kid inside all of us.

While on our camping trip, we always make a canoe trip out to an island that has become known as "Blueberry Island" because of the wild Blueberries that grow there. On one of our first trips to the park, I remember a per-son swimming from shore with a canoe for an escort around the island and then back to shore. I remember thinking to myself at that time that that person must be a lifeguard or a competitive swimmer.

Looking back now that swimmer's round trip was only about one kilometre long. It's remarkable how my perspective has changed. Fast forward five years and that swimmer is now me. I now swim the two kilometre trip to the island while the others take the canoes. This swim is about half of the distance I swim for a full-distance triathlon so of course I swim back at the end of the day. My swimming to the island has completely changed my experience and has planted a seed in the minds of the kids as they grow older. Last summer my son Warren who was seventeen at the time joined me for the swim out to the island. Being active is a great way to demonstrate leadership by example. If I had never swum to the island, my son would not have tried it and we would not have had that experience together.

Now that Warren is in his second year at University, whenever I want to inspire him to do more than practicing to be a sloth like so many university students are doing, I reminisce about that swim and I like to remind him that while I'm getting faster with age, his new social habits and lack of exercise are slowing him down. I try very hard not to tell him what to do. I simply present him with options. I have to trust he is smart enough to make the best decisions.

I think running has always been my favorite of the three activities in the park. Where we camp, we are about six kilometers from the main interior launching point for canoe trips into the park interior. There you will find the

Portage Store, a landmark restaurant, canoe rental centre, and general store for park inhabitants. The summer weather is always hot and humid so it is awesome running to the Portage Store Docks, peeling off everything but the running shorts, jumping in for a quick refreshing dip and then getting out just as fast, putting the running shoes and hat back on and leaving just as quick as you got there. There are always lots of tourists on hand taking pictures and it has just become something of a funny ritual watching those taking pictures of me.

I usually have company on most of my runs now and one of the older boys in his early twenties was just starting to get into running. When I found out he was planning on going for a run in the morning, we set our clocks and planned our running date. We did a 12k run that first day together and while I knew the distance; he had no clue how far I would take him.

The interesting thing about your belief system is that you and the people around you are what set your limits. He had only run as far as 7k and he had his doubts about tackling 12k so I just didn't bother telling him that's how far it was until the run was over. Now that he knows he can run 12k, what

else might he believe he can do? You really
are a product of your environment so if your
immediate environment is unsupportive of
your new heart healthy lifestyle, don't tell
people what you're going to do because they
will only bring you down. Instead, just quietly go about your business and do what you
want to do and just like the pied piper, people will start to follow. This is a great time
to ask the question, "Who will you inspire?"

Your journey will be very personal to you
and the experiences you have will be the
stuff you tell your grandkids about. Your
grandkids won't care about the year you
made your best sales, or the year your job
was the hardest or the year you spent the
summer killing it on a video game. By the
time your kids grow up, video games will be
a thing of the past if they learn how to be active outside. Sure you were an epic video
game player in your day but who really
cares what your high score was in Donkey
Kong? What people will talk about as they
grow older and tell their kids about are the
times grandpa taught us how to canoe and
then he swam to the island while we provided the canoe escort. That same lake will
be there 100 years from now and a new generation will be creating their own memories
and experiences. Just think of the legacy you

could leave for them, one of health, happiness, and filled with rich experiences.

One of the activities I enjoy the most and I learned this at an early age from my dad was how to make home movies. While the days of projectors, screens, and film reels are long gone, I enjoy documenting my experiences on YouTube because that is my channel to showcase my experiences to the world. My videos are public and you can see everything from my races to swimming in Algonquin Park on my YouTube channel. Videos are a really cool way to express yourself and share you story. Looking back now, if you listen to the music selections, they typically give you my frame of mind at the time. It's a fun transition to watch unfold.

So as you start or continue on with your own journey, think about how heart healthy activity can become part of your everyday life no matter where you find yourself in the world. When I travel on vacation, I can go online and measure the distance of any beach in the world and know how far my run will be before I even get there. Work these types of challenges into your daily plan.

There is more world out there for you to experience so make the decision to start your
heart healthy journey today and patiently
watch your new life and new outcomes unfold.

Paying it Forward

What's old is new again. The phrase "pay it forward" was coined about 100 years ago, but it's an old concept. Now a new generation has started to embrace it. "Paying it forward" is when the beneficiary of a good deed repays it to others instead of to the original benefactor.

You could say that my chance encounter with a triathlete, and that person's willingness to take the time to talk with a complete stranger for five minutes was repaying a debt to the person who turned him onto the sport of triathlon. It's about doing a good deed in the hopes that the momentum of good deeds will continue to build. His good deed inspired me and now I have inspired over 2000 people and counting. How many people will those people, including you, inspire? The possibility of taking this heart healthy message around the globe is inspiring.

Today, when someone puts a video onto YouTube, it has the potential to be immediately shared by millions of people around the world and when this happens the video is said to have gone "viral". Viral videos rely on "hooks" which draw the audience in to watch them. What kind of "hook" do you need to have to give life to a viral message on the internet? Nobody can predict the answer to that question for sure but here are some surprising numbers. It only takes one person sharing a link with two friends and that process repeating thirty times to have 1 billion unique views of a video on YouTube.

We've witnessed viral videos happen with pop culture music videos. It is possible to reach others with content that is a little more substantial and meaningful in the same way. If someone shared something meaningful with you, would you share it with two friends? I'm not talking about a chain email that you just send to all of your contacts, I'm talking about sharing links to videos that have the potential to change people's lives.

We all have the potential to "pay it forward" by inspiring others with our own stories of success. It might take you a little out of your comfort zone to reach out to others but in order to innovate and make a difference in the world, we have to make ourselves a little uncomfortable at times. Fear and pain are part of the pathway to success.

In my spin class, I don't really enjoy people facing me and hanging on my every move. I would rather have my back to the group and just ask them to follow my lead. As uncomfortable as I might feel being at the focal point of the class, facing the group gives me the opportunity to view everyone with a coach's eye. I see my role as an instructor as being more of a coach with the purpose of helping others. I don't go to spin class for my own workout, I go to help inspire others to get the most out of their valuable time. I find my reward in paying forward the investment that others have taken in my life.

Who could you inspire? Will you inspire your friends, your co-workers, your neighbors or even your family? Will you inspire a complete stranger who asks you a simple question?

Paying it forward can be as simple as smiling more because when you smile, you feel better about yourself and that makes others around you feel good too. When you feel good about yourself, you project it in many ways and it rubs off on everyone around you. Remember my old boss, Rick? He was a strong leader. He taught me the value of a simple smile and how impactful that can be. While I haven't seen Rick in years, I know that he made a strong impression on me. Now I am paying it forward by smiling more and making others feel good about themselves in the process. While teaching at my cycling studio tonight, I made a point of greeting everyone by their first name as they entered the studio. At some point during the class as I was making my rounds around the room I had an opportunity to get everyone smiling. All of the problems of the day just seemed to melt away if only for those forty-five minutes. The simple act of people smiling together as a community has the capacity to change our moods, our minds, and our outlook on life.

Who Will You Inspire?

I have always believed that there is greatness within each and every one of us, and
this is your time to shine!

Don't ask, "What do you want to be?" Ask,
"Who do you want to be?" What legacy do
you want to leave? What will you be remembered for most?" These are not simple
questions and definitely there are no easy
answers. If you want to be described or remembered as a fun, loving and inspired human being, then live every day starting today as a fun, loving and inspired human being.

As for me, I have believed from a very early
age that my purpose here on earth was to inspire and help serve other people. When I
was a young boy, I would often go up to the
podium after church service and look out
over an empty crowd. Someone once asked
me if I wanted to be a minister one day and I
replied no. Back then, I just liked the idea of
people looking up to me. It has taken me
half a lifetime to figure out what I was going
to be when I grow up and what I am is a
husband, father, coach, athlete and entrepreneur. Who I am is a leader. I live my life in a

way that I believe others can easily follow. It is a very rewarding and fulfilling feeling knowing that my purpose in life is to help serve and inspire other people to experience living heart healthy lives.

If only one person doesn't have to suffer through a life riddled by heart disease or learns how to manage their weight because they read this book and were inspired to make the necessary changes, then I will have lived my life being the person who I was meant to be.

There are millions of books in print right now. Some will sell millions of copies while others might be lucky just to sell only a few. When I started on this journey, it was never about selling books. It was about taking care of myself so I will be around for my family and in the process show my friends and neighbors that a balanced lifestyle far out-weighs any other alternative.

The beauty of the information age is that knowledge is inexpensive, empowering, and easy to obtain. We all have the ability to make real and lasting change in our lives by gaining a fresh new perspective. Only you can choose what information is right or wrong for you because ultimately you will be living with the outcome.

One of the biggest problems with copious amounts of information is knowing what to do with it once you have it. Over the years, I have attended many seminars and motivational workshops and the biggest problem with those delivery models is putting the information into practice once you get home. I don't want that to be a problem for you and that is why I created www.heartfit365.com. The purpose of this website is to provide you with the specific information you need to succeed. You will also find inspiration and motivation that will support you and keep you on track every day, further helping you to reach and attain your goals.

While I don't believe that any one true heart healthy exercise program is better than another one, I do believe that once you understand what your body needs to reach your goals, you will be able to enjoy your favorite fitness activities with a renewed sense of purpose.

What I hope you will take away from this book is a common sense understanding of how your body and mind either works for you or against you to reach your goals every day. You should also be informed enough now to ask your fitness provider the right questions so that you can make the best choices for the life you want to live.

So I ask you: who are you going to be, and who will you inspire? What new perspective have you gained about the choices you've been making? Is your old way of doing things working for you or do you need a new plan? Have you achieved your desired outcome for your life? If you have made it this far through my book, I sincerely believe you would like to experience something more.

I have one simple request. If this book inspires you to live your life in a healthier way than you are currently living, reach out and share your story with me online at www.heartfit365.com. Twenty years from now (2035), if you pass another age group athlete in any kind of race and he has 68 marked on his right calf right, please be sure to say hello, it just might be me. In any case, you will make that person's day just by saying "keep up the great work, you're doing awesome".

Just a side note about social media: some
people spend hours every day on social media when they could be spending time investing in themselves. I like social media for
one simple reason; it can help you connect
or reconnect with people in a very positive
way. I have a friend named Mike who I went
to elementary school with and when high
school came we parted ways going to different schools. About five years ago we con-
nected again through social media. Mike had
moved to Florida many years ago and we
hadn't seen each other in about 35 years. He
was following my triathlon journey through
my social media pages and we had recon-
nected with a few short emails. Last summer, he was in my home town visiting his
mom when I literally bumped into him at a
store. We chatted for a couple minutes and
he congratulated me on my triathlon accomplishments. He told me he had just under-
gone a kidney transplant, donated from his
brother about a year ago and that he was
well onto his road to recovery. About four
months ago, I received another message
from Mike. Through the example I had set
and with his doctor's clearance, he decided
that he was going to take full advantage of
his new lease on life and that he wanted to
try this triathlon thing too. Since that email,
we have picked up our friendship right

where it left off and we are like two kids in a candy store who can talk endlessly about triathlon. I have been coaching him, just like I want to help coach you through my online coaching videos. We've exchanged several fun emails and phone calls about buying swim, bike, and run equipment, and training. It is so rewarding to know that the example you set and the life you lead has had an impact that goes beyond your own benefits and reaches out and touches the lives of people who you know and care about.

Thank you for taking the time to read about my story. If my experiences can help to change your life for the better, then all of my work and coaching will have been worthwhile.

The only question left to ask is: *Who will you inspire?*

So you've come this far, you've read the entire book...now what?

First, visit my website www.heartfit365.com and sign up for FREE to become a member of our community. Next, take a look around the website at the videos and information I have posted to help you gain new perspective. Check out the learning page where I have posted a FREE video about looking good, feeling good and inspiring others.

If journaling is your thing, create a free account on www.myfitnesspal.com and start tracking your daily physical activity and food consumption. If you are using a heart rate monitor, you will want to make sure the calories burned from exercise are recorded from your heart rate monitor and not automatically populated from the website. A few incorrect calories may not seem like much but they can make all the difference if you are trying to manage your expectations for weight management.

Finally, if you want more support, coaching and inspiration, consider hosting a Heartfit365 Workshop in your community or your place of work. I will personally come and answer all of the questions that are most important to you. You can find out more information about hosting a workshop from our website on the WORKSHOP page.

Could someone you know benefit from reading Heartfit365? It's the perfect gift for parents in their 40s who want to experience a healthier outcome for their life. You can order a copy of Heartfit365 from Amazon.com, obtain a copy through one of my Heartfit365 Workshops or by ordering it directly from the Heartfit365.com website.

To get your own Heartfit365 silicone glow in the dark wrist band that reads PERSPECTIVE – CHOICES – OUTCOME, simply attend one of my seminars or workshops and receive one for free.

Final thoughts…*Your kids will be who you are so be the person you want them to be.*

www.ingramcontent.com/pod-product-compliance
Lightning Source LLC
Chambersburg PA
CBHW030436290526

45786CB00001B/319